A better world for children?

Current debates about children only rarely go beyond an elabora-
tion of those familiar headlines – sexual abuse, violence against
children, youth crime, the damaging effects of divorce and the
failures of social work and of parenting. Michael King now takes
these and other emotive issues about children as the starting point
for a highly original, wide-ranging analysis of decision-making, pol-
icy-formulation and moral campaigns aimed at improving the world
for children. In a truly interdisciplinary work he uses the sociological theory of self-referential systems to examine how what today
constitutes truth and valid knowledge in our society has become
fragmented with science, law, politics, and economics operating as
distinct and often conflicting sites of authority

This fundamental change in the nature of society, he argues, has
devastating effects for the optimistic principle which inspired so
many past reforms – the belief that personal morality may be galva-
nized into social action through changing attitudes and altering
interpersonal behaviour. Today the only way forward is through a
radical reconceptualization of social problems to take account of
this change, even to the point of revising our understanding of what
we mean by 'society'.

This is a critical and challenging book. It should be read by all
those with an interest in social policy in general and, in particular,
policies aimed specifically at improving children's lives.

Michael King is Professor and Co-Director of the Centre for the
Study of Law, the Child and the Family at Brunel University.

A better world for children?

Explorations in morality and authority

Michael King

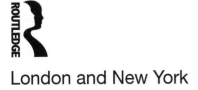

London and New York

First published 1997
by Routledge
2 Park Square, Milton Park, Abingdon, Oxon, OX14 4RN

Simultaneously published in the USA and Canada
by Routledge
270 Madison Ave, New York NY 10016

Transferred to Digital Printing 2007

© 1997 Michael King

Typeset in Times by Routledge

British Library Cataloguing in Publication Data
A catalogue record for this book is available from the British Library

Library of Congress Cataloguing in Publication Data
King, Michael, 1942
  A better world for children? : explorations in morality and authority /
Michael King.
  p. cm.
Includes bibliographical references and index.
  1. Child welfare. 2. Social systems. 3. Autopoiesis. 4. Ethics.
I. Title.
HV713 K555 1997   96–32311
362.7–dc20   CIP

ISBN 0–415–15017–5 (hbk)
ISBN 0–415–15018–3 (pbk)

Contents

Preface

This has not been an easy book to write. Not that any enterprise based on the theory of autopoietic systems could ever be easy. To start with, one never knows where to start, for wherever one begins, it is always the middle. Autopoietic theory contains a total theory of society in a way that makes it impossible to detach one part of the theory and examine it in isolation from the whole. Yet to devote a major chunk of a book about children to providing a full account of this scheme would be unfair to those readers who are not particularly interested in the complexities of social theory. Second, I was aware that wherever I began this book, it would in the eyes of many sociologists and almost all lawyers and social workers, be the wrong place. Traditionally (one could almost say 'intuitively') any discussion of children begins with families and, if not with families, then at least with people. To ask readers who have taken the trouble to buy or borrow a book with the word 'children' in the title to abandon the idea that the only social units which have any importance at all are the individual and the family (which consists of a closely knit group of individuals) is like trying to convince soccer fans that the game would be more interesting if played with a square ball.

A third problem is that the approach of autopoietic theory to society and social issues not only breaks with an individualist tradition which has become second nature to most people, but it is also seen as anti-humanist, in the sense that it abandons humanist ideals and aspirations by regarding them as irrelevant to the sociological enterprise. Niklas Luhmann is by no means the first social theorist to take this stance. Another twentieth-century example is Michel Foucault, but at least the vague and at times contradictory nature of Foucault's writings has left the way open for interpreters to claim his support (wrongly I would argue) for the oppressed and exploited sections of humanity. Autopoietic theory, however, is not amenable to such humane misinterpretations. Indeed, where it is misinterpreted, it is usually in the opposite direction. As Luhmann himself acknowledged on a recent visit to London, he is seen as 'the devil', as the arch-sceptic (or arch-conservative) who scoffs at all attempts to make the world a better place. Not surprisingly, this alienates entirely the progressive humanists, those people who want to feel up-beat about the progress made so far in improving the human condition and optimistic about the possibility of even greater progress in the future. Even worse, it provokes the wrath of radical ideologists, whether they be Marxist, feminist, ecologist, communitarians, Thatcherites or new republicans. On the principle of 'who is not for me must be against me', Luhmann and autopoiesis become 'the enemy'.

I was very conscious, while writing this book, that by not actively supporting either progressive humanist or critical ideologist accounts of the way forward for children, I might well, like Luhmann, find myself branded as 'the enemy', particularly by children's rights activists, legal positivists, social welfarists and radical feminists. It is certainly true that throughout the book I point to the limitations of their particular perspectives and reveal my own worries about the claims and ambitions of their supporters. Yet I do not think that this should make me their enemy. My lack of commitment to these positions certainly does not indicate any hostility on my part but rather the detachment of a sociological observer. I am only too aware that, according to some versions of sociology, there can be no such thing as detachment and that any statement about social issues is an expression, whether overt or covert, of a political ideology. I am also aware that, for these and other sociologies, sociological observation only has value if it can be translated directly into social action – today's research results or sociological insights are tomorrow's data for effective decision making. These are both positions which I reject for reasons which will become apparent in the chapters of the book.

Returning to the difficulties which I experienced in writing this book, these were in part, as I have explained, inherent in the nature of the task of applying the theory of autopoiesis to an area of social concern which, since Nietzsche in 1882 announced the death of God, has until the arrival of postmodernism, been monopolized by humanists, progressivists (whether Whig or Fabian), legalists and radical utopian thinkers. The way that I chose to circumvent the problem of reconciling the irreconcilable was, at the very start, to set them up in opposition to one another. This takes the form of a dialogue in Chapter 1 between moral philosophy as adopted by the would-be protectors of children and preventers of harm against them, and the observers of their moral and regulatory efforts, who are the autopoieticists. This is not totally satisfactory, but at least it indicates in a simple and direct way a break with traditional ways of seeing child welfare issues and so sets the theoretical tone for the six chapters on substantive issues which form the core of the book.

The other difficulty which I finally need to mention concerns the origins of the book. As will no doubt become apparent, four of the chapters began life as separate essays. Each was written at a different time and at a different stage in my own understanding and appreciation of autopoietic theory. The earliest of these is Chapter 3 which focuses on and is critical of the law's construction of child abuse. This was written at a time when my attitude towards the legal system was probably closer to that of Habermasian commitment than to Luhmannian agnosticism. Today, I would be less confident that social scientific analyses of the Cleveland and Orkney child abuse fiascoes would have been better in any absolute sense than those attempts to create a new order which Lords Butler-Sloss and Clyde offered in their reports. They would certainly have been different. These differences between social scientific accounts and those produced by lawyers in their attempts to reconstitute moral agendas as legal issues are identified in Chapter 5, which deals with the James Bulger trial and its aftermath.

Finally, I would not want readers to start this book with the impression that the articles have been randomly thrown together and, therefore, can be read in any order without loss to coherence. While Chapter 1 is clearly an introduction and Chapter 8 clearly a conclusion the order of the inner chapters does represent an attempt to develop a major theme of the book, that of the impossibility of directly changing society in preferred ways by altering individual consciousness. While direct translations from the moral to the social may once have been possible, the nature of modern society, with its functionally differentiated, closed but interdependent systems, means that changes in society can take effect only through the medium of social communications. The effects of these communications are even more difficult to predict than those of moral communications on individual consciousness. This theme comes to the surface in Chapters 2, 4, 6 and 7, which deal with the efforts of social workers to act morally and the attempts of anti-child abuse campaigners and international children's rights activists to impose a moral order on an unruly world. I wish that I could add that the book becomes increasingly optimistic. If this is not possible then at least, after the bleakness of the earlier chapters, the final chapter does offer some glimpses of light and hope, if only to sociologists.

Michael King
London, May 1996

Acknowledgements

I should like to express my warm thanks to my colleagues at the Centre for the Study of Law, the Child and the Family, Alison Diduck, Felicity Kaganas and Christine Piper, for their support and encouragement throughout the time when I was struggling with this book and for their comments on and corrections to the many draft chapters of this book. For non-autopoieticists their tolerance has been quite remarkable. I should also like to thank David Bradley, Jean Floud, Patrick Parkinson and Anton Schütz who have spent more time than I could possibly have expected reading my efforts and commenting on the inadequacies of my theoretical ideas and my attempts to apply them to concerns about children. If the final version of the book is now much stronger and more coherent than it was in draft form, then this is due in no small part to their efforts. Finally, I should like to express my gratitude to the editors and publishers of *The Journal of Social Policy*, *Soziale Systeme*, *The International Journal of Children's Rights* and *Acta Juridica* for allowing me to republish the articles which form the main part of Chapters 3, 4, 5 and 7 of this book.

An earlier version of Chapter 3 originally appeared in *The Journal of Social Policy* under the title 'Law's Healing of Children's Hearings. The Paradox moves North'. Similarly, Chapter 5 is a reworking of an article which originally appeared in *The International Journal of Children's Rights* under the title, 'The James Bulger Murder Trial: Moral Dilemmas and Social Solutions' and Chapter 4, of an article which was published in the German journal, *Soziale Systeme*, under the title of *Managerialism versus Virtue. The Phoney War for the Soul of Social Work*. Finally, an earlier version of Chapter 7 appeared recently in the South African journal, *Acta Juridica* under the title, 'Against Children's Rights'.

Chapter 1

Good intentions into social action

MORALITY

Little in life arouses moral indignation and demands moral judgments and action more than the suffering of children, so let us start
this book with morality and the ways we distinguish between good
and evil. Moral discourses take the spectacle of children's suffering
and seek out the evil that has caused that suffering. In a powerful
symbolic way the suffering of children comes to represent the
exploitation of the powerless, the abuse of the defenceless, innocence defiled. The relief of this suffering, the banishment of evil,
the restoration of good, becomes a moral campaign for which children symbolize virtue, innocence and powerlessness. Children
become symbols of the good which needs to be protected against
the powerful, against evil – the abusers, molesters, batterers,
exploiters, who treat children in selfish, callous, indifferent, cruel
ways. Children must also be protected against the imperfect world
that adults have created with its dangers, its pollutants, its inequalities, its injustices. Children's suffering inspires moral campaigns to
combat what comes to be seen as 'abuse', to rescue children from it,
to protect them from it and prevent it and to punish those who continue to perpetrate it.[1] 'Abuse' itself comes to represent an evil
which can eventually be defeated through concerted efforts on the
part of the social forces of good, the task becomes one of rooting
out the causes of this evil and systematically eliminating them, predicting where the next outbreak will occur, and making anticipatory
strikes, identifying victims in advance and moving them metaphorically, and in some cases, literally to safer ground.

Once the evil that causes children's suffering has been renamed
'abuse', the way lies open for different forms of action to expose

abuse and combat it and its effects. This action may take a social hygienic form, where abuse is seen as endemic in those parts of society which lack such healthy attributes as community spirit, neighbourliness, a social conscience, parenting skills, self-discipline, religion and education as would immunize them against evils. They may take on the medical form of diagnosing pathologies to be remedied through therapy and treatment of the biological or psychological symptoms or underlying causes of the aberrant behaviour. Recently, they have taken on the form of classifying certain families as 'dysfunctional' and of correcting the malfunctioning through various kinds of remedial treatment. All these campaigns against abuse are founded on the notion of intervention, interfering with the relationship between the abused and the abuser, or changing the conditions that are seen to give rise to the abuse. Such intervention is authorized by such powerful moral justifications as 'the needs of the child' , 'children's welfare' or 'the interests of the child'. Although, as we shall see, in order to achieve social authority these moral actions have usually to be supported today by medical or scientific evidence.

A very different form that moral campaigns take begins with the spectacle of the vulnerability and powerlessness of children. Here children's suffering is seen as the result of this powerlessness (or the powerlessness of those who wish to protect or rescue them) and the advantage taken of that powerlessness by adults who dominate and exploit them or act in ways that are indifferent to their needs and interests. This moral campaign has taken the form of giving children 'rights', that is, rights of autonomy which oblige adults to regard them as people rather than objects, of arming them with the power to say 'no' and to make known what they want so that other adults may help them to achieve these ends. In this way they, or those authorized to interpret what they want or need, will be better able to defend themselves against the harms perpetrated upon them by adults and the adult world. Rights, therefore, not only represent power in the hands of the rights-holder, but they also force others to treat the rights-holder with respect. As one author wrote recently of children's rights, 'giving rights to children is . . . a public and palpable acknowledgement of their status and worth' (Archard, 1993, p.168–169).

Moral principles into social action

If the immediate responses against child abuse are to move beyond the stage of emotional reactions and serve as a springboard for campaigns to protect and relieve the suffering of children, there has first to be some consolidation of these responses around acceptable moral principles. Second, practical measures have to be devised for changing people's behaviour towards children.

For the first of these requirements, philosophers are at hand to remind us that society's treatment of children is not merely a matter of early intervention, practical reasoning and skilful prediction. There are issues of principles and values at stake, which need to be resolved by society, before policies can be drafted and decisions made. Moral philosophy occupies itself specifically with the analysis of moral tenets – what constitutes virtue and vice and how these distinctions are morally justified.[2] Yet moral philosophers do not confine themselves to the analysis of the values contained in codes for good and evil, morality and immorality. They are also, and perhaps even principally, concerned with showing how these codes can be improved so as to serve as guidelines for 'practical action', for the encouragement of moral behaviour and for the discouragement of immorality. Here moral philosophy often merges with political philosophy in attempting both to set out for society a set of moral objectives, and indicating the possible ways of achieving these objectives through different forms of social organization. Much of the theoretical writing on children's rights is of this nature. Political philosophy assists in a general understanding of the ways that moral values may become deployed in society. While they are not directly concerned with practical issues such as the drafting and enforcement of laws, they attempt to analyse political institutions and to propose the kind of political order that would be necessary for moral principles to find expression in practical action. These may be related to such matters as the role of the state, the family, education, the class structure or the deployment of legal and other regulatory measures, such as distributions of wealth and power. At this level of philosophical analysis, the moral campaigns for preventing, and protecting children against, the evil that is child abuse bring together three important concerns (1) debates about what is and what is not in the interests of children, (2) issues around the distinction between children and adults, and (3) problems relating to the division between private and public and more particularly, between the family and the outside world.

This leads to the second requirement, the need for effective practical action. How can society make parents take more responsibility for their children's well-being? How can social workers better intervene at an early stage in situations of risk? How can greater cooperation between all those social agencies concerned with different aspects of children's lives be achieved, to enable more effective and better-informed decisions to be made or to empower children or those that seek to protect them? Issues such as these are the stock-in-trade of policy formulators and decision makers. In seeking to answer these difficult questions they necessarily pass from the level of abstract principles to that of applying practical knowledge. This does not represent an abandonment of morality, but rather the necessity of passing from the abstract paradigm of vice and virtue to the practical world of harm and benefits. This brings into the arena disciplines, such as paediatrics, psychology and psychiatry, pedagogy and nutrition, which in modern society have the task of identifying the kinds of behaviour and environmental conditions that are good for children and those which are likely to harm children. The last fifty years have seen a massive growth, not only in the number of such experts, but also in the width and depth of their expertise. Harms which were once considered as inevitable or matters of fate are now seen as controllable, and the results of decisions or the failure to make the appropriate decisions.

DISAPPOINTED EXPECTATIONS

It is often very difficult to know whether these moral campaigns succeed in achieving their objectives. Of course, where these objectives are very specific, such as raising the level of nutritional intake or the reduction or elimination of certain diseases, success and failure are relatively easy to measure. But here the moral concern has been translatable directly into concern for medical action and the attainment of health targets. Where the target concerns changing social policies towards children, the results are far more difficult to estimate. Some appear to succeed, others not. Some work for a time, but then government policy changes or enthusiasm for them wanes and they stop working so well. Others, which appear to work well, create new problems for children which were not anticipated by the promoters of the campaigns or the policy makers who attempted to convert moral principles into social action.

So is it surprising that, despite our living in a 'golden age' for children's rights, where 187 nations of the world have ratified the *United Nations Convention on the Rights of the Child*, even in the prosperous countries of the West children are still subjected to so many forms of harmful behaviour? Why should this be so in a world which has pledged itself to promote the welfare of children? Why do millions of children still suffer the most serious deprivations? Why are they still being exploited? Why are they still being damaged and their future blighted by the behaviour of adults?

These are troubling questions which cast serious doubt on the efforts of moral campaigners to eliminate abuse and construct a better world for children. Yet far from deterring these campaigners in their efforts to promote the welfare of children, such disappointed expectations tend to act as a spur to greater efforts. Disappointments will often lead to revigorized attempts to succeed, but this time using new techniques, new modes of analysis which are guaranteed to improve efficiency and effectiveness. Past failures tend to be seen and explained away as the result of 'practical problems'. The original objectives are still seen as achievable but, as always, problems arise when you try to put principled policies into practice, and part of the task is to overcome them. These obstacles to success, these 'practical problems' may be identified as, for example, lack of resources or the lack of will to allocate sufficient resources to fund programmes, national interests which stand in the way of child-centred policies, superstition and irrational beliefs based on religion or tradition. Obstructions to progress may also be seen to come from vested commercial interests in things remaining as they are or the difficulty of providing adequate proof in the courts to convict people who harm children. Once these 'practical problems' have been identified, it would seem to be only a matter of time before the obstacles they present can be overcome and the campaigns for improving children's lives be set back on track. However, it rarely seems to work like that. Instead, the obstacles themselves tend to become major areas for study and analysis and the more they are studied the more complex the situation seems to become and the further we seem to be from the original problems and ways of solving them. Things have moved on to reveal that what was once thought to be the important issue is now seen as peripheral, and problems of which we were previously unaware are now shown to be central to any resolution. Why should this be? How can social action for children be made more effective? How can success be guaranteed? How can obstacles and unintended consequences be anticipated in advance and so overcome?

It would be comforting if this book were able to answer these questions by pointing to some magical formula which would dissolve all impediments to the improvement of children's lives. Instead, what it attempts to do is to question the very notion of 'disappointed expectations'. Yet, this in itself may well be a useful exercise, for, if people's expectations are changed, the deployment of their energies and inventiveness may also take different directions. If this and the succeeding chapters are able to show that the disappointed expectations of moral campaigners are in fact products not of a faulty world, but of their own unrealistic notions of what is achievable and how these achievements may be realized, some benefits may yet emerge. Yet, in one respect, the aim of this book is to go much further than that. What it attempts to do is to demonstrate in the various themes and topics covered that these disappointments arise from the insistence on a model of society and its operations *which leads inevitably to disappointments*. This is not a matter of self-delusion in any simple meaning of the term, but results rather from the insistence on certain beliefs about what society consists of, which in turn lead to policies and courses of action based on those beliefs. What this book argues is that if the policies and the actions do not lead to the desired results, this is not because of 'practical problems', but is a consequence of particular readings of modern society and the way that it operates. What it will suggest is that these readings construct not only what appear to be solutions, failures and disappointed expectations, but also the very problems that give rise to them. To take this line of inquiry and question the way that moral issues concerning children are constructed will not itself lead to solutions, but it may lead to interesting reformulations of problems.

What then are the principle characteristics of this model of society which give rise to such hopes for regulation and control of harmful conduct towards children, but also to such disappointments? They can be identified as follows:

1   a continuity between consciousness and the social world;
2   people as the primary agents for all social events;
3   direct input–output relations between social groups and organizations;

4 the possibility of identifying definitive causes.

A continuity between consciousness and the social world

This model of society makes no clear distinction between the attitudes, beliefs, ideas and thoughts that pass through the minds of individual people and their communication to others in ways that have meaning for others or make sense to others. It assumes that society is no more or no less than collective consciousnesses made social. It follows, therefore, that to change society one needs only to change the attitudes and beliefs of people. Philosophical ideas, political ideologies, and moral beliefs which may be powerful forces in altering individuals' attitudes towards children and formulating justifications and explanations for their behaviour in relation to them, may, according to this vision of society, also change society in certain preferred directions.

The converse of this view, which I shall be describing later in this chapter, is that consciousness is quite separate from society. While ideas and ideologies may have the power to change people's attitudes, including their way of seeing the world and their own behaviour – in Michel Foucault's term, with 'the care of the self' (Foucault, 1979) – this should not be confused with changing society.

People as the primary agents for all social events

Society is seen, according to this perspective, as the sum of all those people who exist within its boundaries. Neither it nor the social institutions which are regarded as essential to the operation of society, are any different from the people within them. The unity of society, its common purpose and goals, means the unity of its people. It is their conduct and their decisions in their varied social roles which will determine society's future. When, therefore, one talks of law or politics, what one is really referring to are lawyers and politicians. According to this view, social systems such as law, politics and science have no separate identity from the people who operate them. To change society one needs, therefore, to change people, and to improve society, one needs to improve people's behaviour by applying moral programmes, for example, making them less selfish, less violent, less intolerant, and more generous, kind, altruistic, etc. These changes, according to this approach, will automatically improve the operation of social systems, and in the case of children's interests, will cause them to work in ways that promote and protect those interests. This is not to deny that changing the processes and procedures of institutions may also offer a way forward, but since there is no clear distinction between organizations and the people who operate them, the success or failure of such reforms are seen to depend entirely upon their effects on people. Regulation of social organizations, therefore, is no different from the regulation of the people who belong to these organizations. It consists of putting into places of power and responsibility people who are likely to be virtuous, and devising structures to ensure that these right-minded people fill these positions and continue to act in virtuous ways once they have been appointed.

Direct input–output relations

Just as organizations are seen as people, and groups of people relate to one another in direct ways, so the conduct of organizations is no different from the expression of the sum of the people who run them. Relations between the different organizations of society are therefore seen as operating in a relatively simple and direct manner with information passing from one to the other and the decisions of one having a direct effect on the behaviour of the other. This direct input–output relationship may take different forms, according to the perspective of the particular analysis being applied. Society may be seen, for instance, as involving networks of power relationships between people who represent different points of view and/or different interests. More cynical analysts tend, for example, to see politicians, in particular, using their power to make the courts or social workers, universities or scientists, all dance to their tune. Banks and large corporations may be seen as attempting to control the politicians in ways that ensure that their interests are always served. Different interest groups may combine with one another to change society in ways that increase their power and wealth or to combat what they see as being threats to the existing order (which is often identical to their own vested interests). The global scene in this perspective is simply an international version of the same game. The only difference is that people are now representatives of different nations or multinational corporations. One finds here the same conception of action to change things for the better as depending upon strategies, alliances, motivation and rational assessments of gains and losses, and the same notion of a direct relationship between policies and actions. The only difference is that these ways of understanding now take on a global or international dimension.

Other, perhaps more optimistic versions, would see the forces of regulation and control as exercising a restraining and salutary influence on what would otherwise be a chaotic, unjust world, but always in a direct, uncomplex way. The police, judges and lawyers, for example, are portrayed as rooting out corruption and abuses of power in political and financial institutions. Once again, however, the relations are between people who represent (and may be representative of) different social organizations. This is of course the stuff of the culture of films, novels and television dramas, but these fictional representations succeed in attracting a large readership and audience because they rely unquestioningly upon a version of how society works which most people believe, or want to believe, to be true. Furthermore, there is no real difference between these fictional representations and the accounts of national and international events in the news reporting of newspapers and the broadcasting media. Both emphasize the individual, or groups of like-minded individuals, as the prime movers, whether for good or evil, for progress or resistance to progress, in the social world. It is their behaviour which is seen as having a direct impact on history and on the future. Changing organizations is seen as the equivalent of changing people. Organizations are attributed with the same characteristics as people, both good and evil.

The possibility of identifying definitive causes

The assumption that the causes of events in the social world are either self-evident or are out there waiting to be uncovered, is a prerequisite for this model of society. This does not mean that everyone will agree about causes. On the contrary, several different explanations may exist for the same event. People cause harm to children because they are inherently evil, because they have no sense of responsibility, because of their own childhood experiences, because they have not been properly educated in child care, because of stress in their lives. Each of these causal explanations is capable of producing its own kind of regulatory measures, for instance, imprisonment, counselling, therapy, improved living conditions, help in times of crisis, educational courses, or surveillance by social workers.

Failures in regulation are likely to be interpreted in ways which do not usually disqualify the original explanation for the behaviour, but are more likely to cast doubt on the efficiency of those responsible for carrying out the regulatory measures (Howitt, 1992). In a similar manner, apparent successes of regulatory measures based on one causal account do not necessarily invalidate alternative accounts. The continued belief that it is still possible to identify 'the real causes' of harm to children is essential to the notion that such harms are preventable and controllable – whether they consist of a single action by an individual, such as a blow struck in anger which injures a child, or a collective action such as government policies which create 'an underclass', living in pockets of poverty and deprivation. Even if there is controversy over the causes which analysts identify as valid explanations and even if others analysts prefer different explanations, the belief that the establishment of a true cause or true causes is a possibility is a prerequisite to an assumption that regulatory measures may operate upon people's behaviour and so control or eliminate the causes which analysts have identified. The recognition of causes then allows for the possibility of planning and improvements in control over undesirable behaviour. It also allows for prediction and for decisions to be made on the basis that they are not arbitrary or based on speculation, but depend on the existence of chains of causality which have occurred in the past and are likely to recur in the future.

What happens when the unexpected occurs? What happens, for example, when carefully devised plans to secure a child's future welfare, based on accepted ideas about probable sources of benefits and harms to children, are thwarted by such unanticipated events as serious illness, a traffic accident, winning the lottery, falling in love, becoming pregnant, unexpected redundancy, moving home to another country or another part of the same country, or the sudden death of a family member? Only where the occurrence of the disruptive event and its impact on the child and that child's carers were specifically included in the causal account which formed the basis for the prediction will these plans still be likely to hold good. Yet, in practice, when it comes to decisions about helping and protecting children the possibility of unforeseeable occurrences, however common they may be in practice, are unlikely to be included in the evaluation of what is best for the child, simply because they are unforeseeable. By their very nature these events were unpredictable before the decision to adopt the plan, and after the decision they may continue to be seen as chance happenings, which could not have been anticipated and therefore are not to be included in any future exercise in identifying and preventing causes, which may continue unaffected by them. Alternatively, it may be decided that the occurrence of these events should have been foreseen, in which case there may be demands for more detailed and more inclusive causal accounts, so that by including in future the possibility of these events occurring, the accuracy of prediction will be increased. Yet neither the identification of unforeseen causes nor increases in the complexity and scope of causal accounts are likely to prevent the unexpected occurring in future. The problem is not that the particular causal account failed, but that any model which produces the possibility of a definitive account of causality has insuperable problems.

REGULATION AND AUTHORITY WITHIN A CONSTRUCTED WORLD

It is easy to be critical of people who over-simplify and attempt to foist upon us solutions based on simplistic and reductionist solutions, but this is not the purpose either of the preceding section, or of the book as a whole. An alternative approach is to see reduction and simplification as a necessary precursor to any formulation of problems and thus to any proposed solution to those problems. If we take this view it becomes possible to see moral reformers' version of society as consisting of people, or rather of a collective consciousness, to view social organizations as behaving like people and causes as being identifiable as the results of the behaviour of people, not as mistaken, but as *correct in their own terms*, as inevitable if one starts with the formulation of social problems as moral defects.

In order to make this kind of observation we need to pass from a sociology which sees the social world as a factual entity to one which regards all claims to make sense of the world as no more than attempts to give meaning to events which have no intrinsic meaning; meanings are possible only where they emerge out of interpretations. We need to move from a version of social problem-solving which offers the prospect of creating order from a disordered, defective world, to one which observes and attempts to give some meaning to these efforts.

From the perspective of a sociological observer of moral campaigns to improve the defective world, the hopelessness of many such enterprises may appear obvious, but to those engaged in day-to-day problem-solving exercises it may take an appearance similar to that of reassembling the jumbled pieces of a jigsaw puzzle. They may remove each of the pieces from the board to be examined separately from the whole. Then, where pieces are found to be defective, they may perhaps reshape them slightly so as to produce a better fit and put them in their proper place. Once the reformed world is intact, there may be difficulties in keeping the pieces in place, as the social world tends to be shaken about from time to time. But what is needed is social cohesion, to be found perhaps in the law, community spirit, a sense of social responsibility, a willingness to compromise, or good common sense and commitment to progress – which, like super glue, will be guaranteed to keep the pieces in their proper place. Once firmly in place, all the pieces, the elements of the social world, can be relied upon to contribute to the assurance of a secure, happy future.

It was this style of problem-solving that led to the *United Nations Convention on the Rights of the Child*. The problem to be solved here was the suffering and impotence of children throughout the world; the pieces of the jigsaw puzzle were the nations of the world, many of which were seen as pursuing policies and permitting practices that were harmful to children's interests. These defects could be remedied by sensible reshaping. Rules and principles could be produced which would act as guidelines for all future treatment of children in the world, and the combination of law and public opinion would operate as the glue to keep it all together.

Few contemporary sociologists, one should emphasize, would see the social world or society's problems in this unproblematic way. Rather, contemporary social theories, whether postmodernist or poststructuralist, would be likely to question whether the notion that a thing called 'the social world' or 'society' exists as an object to be dissected, manipulated, shaped and improved. Instead what they would propose is that such concepts only have meaning because they become formulated in people's minds and as part of individual or collective interpretations of external events. Society for them is a construct, the meaning of which depends upon the values, beliefs and interpretations of whoever is attempting to make sense of these events.

Once it becomes necessary to regard society or the social world not as an object, but as a construct, a collective abstraction which helps people to make sense of the past, exist in the present and plan for the future, it follows that there may exist not one but many different notions about what society consists of, what makes it work well or what causes it to malfunction. Furthermore, it becomes inevitable that programmes for reform, whether global, national or institutional, will be dependent upon the acceptance of one particular version of what society is – the version which makes it appear that such reforms are possible.

Similarly, recognition of this constructed nature of society and the existence of multiple versions of social reality changes fundamentally the way that a sociological observer would view moral campaigns for improving the world or guarding against undesirable changes to that world. From their perspective, the task of regulating and controlling the future will no longer be seen simply as one of working to a particular blueprint to mobilize the forces of change or overcome the obstacles to change. In addition, part of that task will also include creating a convincing impression that there is indeed 'a society' that is common to everyone, whether it is called 'society' or 'the community', 'our country', 'our world' 'the common good' or 'our culture', so that this entity, this 'something' which the would-be regulators have constructed, can be seen as capable of control in the ways that they have devised. In relation specifically to children, it may be necessary, in order to avoid, eliminate or reduce the risks in situations which are seen as damaging to children, to make people believe that they are part of the same collectivity – be it 'the extended family', 'the nation' or 'the community', be it Europe, the West or the global village – which has common interests and the common objectives of improving children's wellbeing and meeting their needs, which are achievable by working together. Once this notion of collectivity, of consensual interests has been established it may, of course, be reinforced by reference, for example, to 'family values' 'the views of society', 'the interests of society' or 'the common interest' in ways that help to reinforce the belief that this unity actually exists as an object and that it is the power of human action that will change it for better or for worse.

A major problem for moral campaigns today is that of establishing authority for their particular view or construction of society, for without such authority there can be little chance of achieving either the concerted action against harm and abuse or the consensus or 'sense of community' on which such collective action depends.

Determining where today's morality resides is the first problem facing such campaigns. There was a time when religion was able to provide the overriding authority both for the existence of society and the code of conduct that was thought necessary to make that society virtuous. Morality at that time consisted of obeying what were accepted as the laws or commands of a deity or deities who existed beyond the reach of human action. People could affect the behaviour of God or the gods only indirectly, by, for example, making sacrifices or obeying His or their commandments.

Later, when religious authority declined in its effectiveness, moral campaigns were able to rely up to a point upon the authority that resided within individual consciences. Now it was the inner voice which dictated not only personal, but also collective, social responsibility. Virtue or vice in society and the world could be seen as the result of people's adherence to or departure from personal moral codes. Where harm and abuse existed, they were the result of defective individuals or faulty decision making by people working within organizations. It is this type of moral authority which justified the model of society examined earlier which makes no clear distinction between consciousness and society. It is a belief in this moral authority which makes possible a version of society where adherence to moral principles offers the guiding light for the maintenance or improvement of children's well-being and failure to respect those principles result in harm and abuse of children. Discipline and altruism are seen as necessary if 'society' is to progress in ways which are recognized consensually as desirable.[3] An important aspect of effective regulation within this model of society becomes, therefore, formulating common goals which are capable of uniting people with very different political and religious beliefs, different interests, different ideologies and different life-styles. The idea of rights for children provides one set of goals on which it may well be possible to secure the nominal support of everyone, or almost everyone, at least where this is seen as meaning the reduction of suffering and the creation of a better life for children.

It is a short step from a society constructed upon a belief in the authority of the individual conscience to one which vests that authority in a collective conscience representing a consensus or agreed minimum standards as to what constitutes good and bad behaviour towards children. Society is now seen as operating under the authority of a rule of law. The existence of laws, or law-like instruments, such as rules, regulations and lists of accepted practices and guidelines, not only provide the necessary authority for social action; they also convey the impression that behaviour may be effectively regulated through enforcing or encouraging obedience to these 'laws'. This will apply whether the behaviour to be regulated is that occurring between members of families, within organizations or within the boundaries of nation states. The only difference is that the precise legal instrument for authoritative regulation will vary according to the particular level of behaviour that it is intended to regulate. Yet the difficulty with a mode of regulating harmful or potentially harmful behaviour to children which depends on legal authority is that it presupposes a society where law is indeed accepted as the supreme moral authority for what is good or bad for children. Those who wish to give this privileged role to law may well be able to construct such a society for themselves, but, as we shall see, in the version of society that will be adopted in the subsequent chapters of this book, there is no guarantee that others will accord the same privileged role to the legal system or to any other form of authority.

A MULTI-AUTHORITY SOCIETY

The fragmentation of authority

The sociological equivalent of the holy grail, or the philosopher's stone, that elusive entity or element that will provide the key to perfection, is some model of society that captures all complexity in the world, some construction which, when subjected to empirical testing will be found to correspond exactly to the world 'as it really is'. Of course, such a model does not and cannot exist, if only because its very construction would change the external world in ways which the model would not be able to predict, so model and external world would be out of phase as soon as this 'super model' of society came into being. As observers of the social world, including all those different versions of society which are able to co-exist, we are in a somewhat better position to deal with at least some of the complexities than those, like moral campaigners, who are obliged by the very task they have set themselves, to commit themselves to one particular source of authority and so to a version of society where it is possible for that authority to operate effectively so as to achieve the campaigners' moral objectives.

A version of modern society which comes rather closer to reflecting some of its complexity is one where not one but several different bodies of knowledge may be used at different times and in different situations to give authority to decisions, understandings, recommendations and other statements. It could be argued that personal beliefs as to what is right and wrong, good or bad, true or false, etc., might represent the sources of such bodies of knowledge, but there are serious problems with a model of society based on this idea. If this were the case, there would be so many different sources of authority that nobody would know which to accept and which to reject. It would be impossible for people even to communicate except in the most trivial ways. Each one would rely on his or her version of truth or justice, right or wrong. They might be able to exchange platitudes about the weather or their health, but it would be quite impossible for them to co-operate on some concerted action or to take any joint decisions. Even if those who shared the same personal beliefs or moral standards were able to get together under the banner of some 'ideology', this would only form an acceptable basis for social authority where there was wide acceptance of that ideology as being right and true. Yet it is quite clear that modern society exists and continues to exist despite enormous differences in people's personal beliefs, whether they be political, religious, moral or whatever. For this to happen, therefore, there must be some other sites of authority which are unrelated to personal beliefs or to the consolidation of personal beliefs into ideologies.

If we turn specifically to the issue of children, how is it possible within modern society to determine what is good and bad for children or even to devise valid ways for deciding this question? It seems an impossible task today because we are supposedly living in a multicultural, pluralist society where different people and different groups of people give expression to different, equally valid values in their up-bringing of children. Yet the fact remains that such decisions are being made all the time. Where then does the authority for such decisions come from?

One obvious answer is that the authority comes, not from the personal beliefs of the people who make decisions or recommendations about what is good or bad for children, but from the status that we accord to certain people who hold particular positions. We may see these people as capable of drawing upon specialist bodies of knowledge such as law, economics or science and it is this knowledge which gives their decisions and recommendations the necessary authority. Alternatively or additionally, their authority may derive from the fact that they have been appointed to particular positions through the authoritative products of some institution, such as legislation from parliament, legal decisions from the courts, or the appointment of examiners from education. These institutions are therefore seen as legitimate bodies for vesting authority in such people. The important point here is that these bodies of knowledge or systems of appointment operate quite independently of the particular people who make decisions or who contribute to their development. Those accounts of what is good or bad for children's interests and what will be good or bad for them in the future – such as court welfare reports, psychiatric assessments, scientific findings, judge's decisions, acts of parliament, or policy papers – which carry authority in modern society, do not today take the form of personal beliefs. In order to be recognized as socially authoritative, their decisions must conform, both in the language in which they are written and the reasoning which led the writers to their conclusions, to expectations derived from the particular body that possesses the authority to make such statements. These are likely to be law, politics, science and economics, but could also in some situations include religion and education. The differences between these different versions of authority that these bodies or systems represent do not reflect variations in personal consciousness or individual moral values, but rather denote distinctions between the social functions that each of them fulfils for society and its operations.

Let us look at a rather far-fetched imaginary example. A judge strongly believes that television soap operas are destroying children's imagination and that consequently parents should be actively discouraged from exposing their children to them. In deciding between the competing claims of parents for their six-year-old boy to reside with them, the judge asks each one in turn how much control they intend to exercise over the child's television viewing. Having heard their answers, he then gives residence of the child to the one who he considers is more likely to restrict the boy's exposure to soap operas. Contrary to what one might expect, the result of such a decision will not be for the law automatically to amend the catalogue of factors that it recognizes as likely to cause harm to a child, and so justify an order to protect that child. Before the law would be able to adopt this judge's views, his or her beliefs, *as law*, in other words, before such beliefs could be given legal authority, there would first have to be some process of transformation from 'personal views' into grounds or justifications for legal change. Excessive exposure to soap operas would have to be officially recognized by courts not only as a possible cause of harm to children, but also as a valid ground for protective measures towards children. This process may take the political form of legislation, a section in a statute which requires courts to recognize the harm, or, alternatively, a court decision which is confirmed on appeal. Once this recognition has been achieved, the knowledge that excessive watching of soap operas may cause harm to children would be applicable in all future cases, until such time as this knowledge is modified or discarded, again through legal operations, the processes by which the law is changed. It will have achieved the authority of the political and legal systems.

An important additional development to the story is that before arriving at any decision the appeal court judges or a parliamentary committee on legislation would take account of any scientific evidence on the effect of soap operas on children. So law and politics in this particular matter would turn to a different form of knowledge and a different procedure which could be relied upon for determinations of what is good and bad for children. Once again this knowledge exists quite independently of the personal beliefs of the individuals, who in their roles of psychologists and psychiatrists provide such evidence.

Let us pause to take stock of the implications of these events for our model of modern society. Here we have a society which depends for its acceptable accounts of what is good or bad for children on statements which are given an authoritative status because the process by which they were reached conforms with the operations and programmes of a particular social system, which is recognized as a site of authority. Neither of these systems can claim to be dominant, in the sense that the authority of one does not preclude the authority of the others.[4] While each of the systems operates according to its own procedures and its own criteria for determining truth, justice, rightness, these systems are nevertheless dependent the one upon the other for the production of authoritative statements. Law, for instance, will depend upon politics producing legislation for it to interpret and adjudicate upon. It will also depend upon science to produce expert evidence and advice on what is scientifically beneficial or harmful to children. Politics will depend upon law to give its legislative acts the authority of the courts. Science will depend on law and politics for recognition of the truths and falsehoods that it reveals and their transformation into social policies and legal decisions. The nature of the relationship between the systems and the authority they offer is both one of autonomous, simultaneous existence and one of interdependence.

One further matter arising from this case needs to be explored. The fact that the court of appeal decided to call upon scientific evidence did not mean that all existing psychological or psychiatric knowledge relating to children's welfare automatically became law. If that had been the case, we should have been back with the direct input–output model that we described earlier. No doubt there exists a wealth of scientific knowledge about a multitude of factors that might adversely or beneficially affect children's development, but only a small proportion of this knowledge finds its way into legal decisions. There may be several reasons that the courts fail to recognize some and not other items of such knowledge, but these reasons are much more likely to be related to concerns of the law than to the scientific status of such knowledge. The harms that they reveal may, for example, be too difficult to prove in court or they may simply not have been raised as an issue in legal proceedings. Similarly, political bodies may chose to ignore certain scientifically proved harms to children, because it would not be politically expedient to draw attention to them or because it would be far too expensive to tackle them. Legal, political or economic recognition of what is scientifically harmful to children will not, therefore, consist of direct translations from the scientific. Instead, these systems will select such scientific knowledge as will have meaning within their own programmes and will reformulate it in ways which allow such knowledge to exist as part of their own operations. The same will, of course, be true of scientific (including sociological) accounts of law, politics and economics. These accounts would also be selections of such features of those systems as are capable of being formulated within scientific theories and research methods.

DECISION MAKING

The selection of explanations

In modern society a multiplicity of explanations exists for the same social event. Where harms to children is concerned, it is no longer possible to point one's finger at one factor or set of factors and say definitively, 'this is the one and only explanation for what happened'. Even the results of official government inquiries, the decisions of courts or scientific research projects, arouse controversy and provoke alternative accounts and explanations drawing upon different attributions of causality. It is not simply that people apply different belief systems in their interpretation of events in the world and, therefore, cannot agree on one version of historical events.

There is not even agreement on what criteria should be applied to determine the truthfulness or validity of different versions. Scientific criteria are not the same as legal proof, which is not the same as political reality. This multiplicity of ways of evaluating possible explanations reflects the fragmentation of functions in modern society and the way in which modern society vests authority simultaneously in several of these systems. The best that society can do today is to produce causes which are recognized as true or probably true, using the interpretive framework of one system, according to that system's own procedures or processes for determining validity.

Where a society is predominantly organized according to the different functional operations that proceed simultaneously alongside one another, as is today's society, the existence of not one but several sites of authority necessarily creates serious problems for social activists who wish to change that society in predetermined directions. These problems arise from the possibility that statements produced using one set of criteria, which society regards as authoritative, may not be able to take into account a whole range of factors which would be recognized as relevant, or even essential, using criteria derived from different sites of authority. As we have seen, a court cannot take into account simultaneously all possible accounts of causality factors. It has to select between them. Any decisions it makes have only to be lawful. It may be blind to political accounts, such as one which identifies the power imbalance between men and women as the crucial factor in child sexual abuse (see Chapter 2). Its members may also close their eyes to scientific notions of what constitutes truth and validity. Once a legal decision has been made based on this selected version of causality, it remains valid as law, even though the rationale for the decision does not conform with what many people believe to be 'the true explanation' or 'a fair outcome'. The same will be the case in the selection of what constitutes relevant or valid evidence for decisions. Economic decisions, for example, will be based on information selected because it has validity within economics or may be easily translatable into factors for economic programmes. One cannot expect a company making an economic decision to close down an unprofitable factory to take account of the effects on the children of people made redundant as a result of the closure. Social scientists may demonstrate a correlation between unemployment and child malnutrition, and paediatricians may prove the existence of a relationship between child malnutrition and performance on intelligence tests, but, unless these findings are reconstructible as economic factors, the company is likely to be blind to them and, despite the possible adverse consequences for children, the decision it makes is still likely to be regarded as good economics.

The existence of system selectivity, the restricted vision of the external environment, including all possible explanations and versions of causality in that environment, represents at one level a retreat from the overwhelming complexities of the modern world into more reassuring, more certain, more controllable ways of organizing the present and predicting the future. Here within the internal, controlled environment of the system, disruptions such as information about gender inequalities or consequences for children's intelligence, are not permitted to penetrate in their original form. They may enter only if the system is able to see them and only after they have been transformed into some form of knowledge or information that can be subjected to that system's operations. This has considerable consequences for the way in which matters of chance and danger enter the system's operations and programmes.

Risks and dangers, chance and foreseeability

In the same way that information from a system's environment may enter a system only upon its transformation into a form that the system is able to recognize, what were once regarded as 'dangers' may come to be perceived as 'risks', if by 'dangers', we refer to 'acts of God', matters of coincidence or chance happenings, and 'risks' is the term used to describe losses which are seen as the result of decisions or the failure to take decisions.[5] By reformulating dangers within the programmes of those systems which society has designated as capable of producing authoritative accounts of causality, these dangers become reconstituted as 'risks'. In relation to the physical abuse of children, what were once, for example, seen as the unlikely results of over-zealous disciplining now are seen as being the consequence of the lack of vigilance on the part of social workers. As each system increases the complexity of its own internal programmes to deal with an increasingly complex social world (itself the product of the increased complexity of other systems), so the scope of what is 'knowable' and so seemingly 'controllable' widens and so risk increases. Risks, unlike dangers, create the expectation that avoidance and reduction of losses, such as harms to children, are possible, since decisions are seen as being the causes of these events. This in itself does not make the world a safer or a more dangerous place for children in any absolute way, but it does mean that it becomes a more 'risky' place both for children and adults and especially for those whose role is to protect children and promote their welfare. Expectations have been raised of the possibility of control through decision making over a wide range of factors that are seen as dangerous for children's well-being. As more and more knowledge is acquired about those factors which affect outcomes for children, so children's lives become increasingly risky (and also dangerous) and the pressures grow for decisions to be made which avoid or minimize these risks. Yet, as we have seen, what is and is not construed as 'risky' depends on the interpretive framework of the decision makers and those observing the performance of the decision makers.

Within organizations there are always pressures to reduce risks, but the selection of what constitutes risk, and what dangers (not attributable to decisions) will be determined by the internal programmes of the organization. Child protection teams, for example, may see the physical abuse of a child as a risk attributable to the team's decision, and the child's mother's emotional devastation following the separation from her abusing partner, as a danger. For family therapists, on the other hand, the mother's emotional collapse and the consequent break-up of the family may be seen as a risk that is attributable to their therapeutic decisions, and the recurrence of the abuse of the child as a danger. Risks, therefore, may be perceived as dangers and dangers as risks. While each organization may attempt to minimize the risks that it recognizes within its programmes and so give the appearance of efficiency and control, they will be blind to those risks that they do not recognize, or may see them only as dangers. The more efficient their operations become in reducing risk, the more extensive may become the categories of events that they perceive as dangers and the risks that these dangers create for other organizations.

In the light of what we now know about modern society and its organization, the distinction between chance factors and 'practical problems', between what events are perceived as controllable and what are accepted as beyond the reach of regulation becomes largely redundant. The designation of 'chance factor' can be applied only to a narrow range of occurrences, such as natural disasters, and even here it is becoming increasingly likely that some blame will be attributed to defects in forecasting or in the technological devices deployed as indicators of impending hurricanes, earthquakes, volcanic eruptions, etc., or the failures of the authorities to clear the area or bring in rescue teams sufficiently quickly. The same is of course the case where disasters to children occur, whether they concern an individual child's death or serious injury or the deaths or suffering of vast numbers of children. What could at one time have been attributed to 'chance factors' are increasingly likely to be seen as 'practical problems'. Campaigns to save, help and protect children are increasingly likely to identify such items as 'human error', 'self-serving attitudes' or 'administrative inefficiencies' as the causes of these events.

Yet the situation may seem very different from the perspective of the decision makers for whom unforeseen occurrences appear to throw off course even the most carefully considered predictions and the best laid plans. Of course, an observer of the decision maker's past performance will always be able to see in retrospect beyond the information that was available at the time the decision was taken. For the observer events were unforeseeable only because of the failure of the minister or the social work team to recognize them as possible future occurrences.

From a safe vantage point an observer will engage in the exercise of identifying those features which distinguish the predictable from the unforeseeable. These are then interpreted as such matters as lack of foresight, defects in the system or misinterpretation of the signs. For the people being observed, however, the demarcation line falls between what can be known and, therefore, possibly brought under control, and what remains unknowable and thus uncontrollable. In their version of reality and causality, in their account of what is knowable, this distinction relates entirely to matters external to the system itself, but occurring in that system's environment. In practice both of these distinctions fail to do justice to the complexity of the situation. Take the example of a decision by a social worker to place a child with long-term foster parents, who appeared from the extensive information collected for the file to have all the positive attributes for promoting that child's future well-being. Yet, shortly after the placement of the child, there was a world economic recession and a collapse of the housing market. As a result both parents lost their jobs, could not pay the accumulated arrears on their mortgage, were eventually evicted and obliged to move to much smaller rented accommodation. They felt unable to continue with the fostering arrangement and returned a by now desolate child to the children's home. How helpful in this situation is the distinction between chance factors and foreseeable problems? Both the recession and the collapse of the housing market were predictable (at least by some economists) but the problem was that what was 'knowable' to social work's programmes did not include economic forecasts. For social workers economic 'risks' were seen as 'dangers'. Yet, the observer of the social work assessment could legitimately argue that, as the result of poor decision making a child was made to suffer the disappointment of a failed fostering – which, according to some psychologists, might affect that child's emotional development for many years to come.

This example raises fundamental questions concerning attempts to plan for the future of children in today's world. If the distinction between chance factors and practical problems can no longer be relied upon to indicate what is and what is not controllable or able to be regulated, being itself a construct of the perspective of the particular observer, how can one believe that it is possible to create a better world for children?

Reformulations of morality

Judging by the multitude of non-governmental organizations that exist and are active throughout the world in promoting the well-being of children in a myriad of different ways, it is clearly still possible to have faith in the creation of a better world. My argument in this book should certainly not be taken as a demand for the abolition or curtailment of the activities of these organizations. It is rather to suggest that they are able to continue in their activities only by presenting to themselves and to the external world a version of society which ignores the complexities, the difficult issues that I have raised in the last few pages. They are able to do so only by remaining at a level of pre-sociological analysis or, using the terminology of systems, to close themselves away within a system which sees the world in terms of personal responsibility, individual conscience, commitment, sacrifice, guilt, and the like. The way that they are able to make these concepts appear to operate at the level of institutional, governmental and global decision making, is to reformulate them in terms which give the impression that such bodies act and think *in identical ways to people* or that should be seen in such a way as if *they consisted only of collections of individuals*, whose personal opinions, hopes, fears, attitudes and beliefs lie behind the formulation of decisions and policies.

Put slightly differently, while the programmes of these child welfare organizations may relate to complex political, legal, economic, educational, scientific and religious issues, the organizations for helping and protecting children are able to make sense of these different spheres of knowledge and activity largely through concepts derived from moral philosophy. Of course, moral philosophy with its codes and principles may also be seen as representing in its own right a distinct system of understanding with its own identity and its own concerns, but, for campaigners for a better world for children, the problem is not, it must be emphasized, how to make people more moral but rather how to translate moral agendas for children into *effective social action*. In attempting such a difficult task society can no longer return to a pre-Marxian epoch where it conceived of itself as collections of individuals or the sum of individual consciousnesses. In modern society what determines the degree of social effectiveness of decisions and actions based on the prospect of change are not those principles, precepts, ideas and convictions of moral or political philosophers. Rather they are exclusively social events, and social events, as we now know, are quite separate from the factors that motivate, inspire and restrain individuals. Moral principles run up against all those obstacles which were identified as preventing a personal belief from becoming an authoritative communication for modern society – for example, scientific processes and truth criteria, political expediency, economic viability and legal rules of procedures and evidence.

This does not mean that campaigns for the acceptance of moral principles are not recognized or have no effect whatsoever within society. It is rather that they can serve only as 'irritants' to social systems. As such those moral principles which campaigners wish to prevail can enter social systems only in a transformed state, that is, only in forms that allow for their reconstruction within each system, that make sense for the system's programmes and operations.

Furthermore, when it comes to authoritative accounts of social events in the modern world the hermeneutics of moral standards for individuals (or groups of individuals) simply do not have the capacity to reformulate or replace social forms of knowledge. While morality insists on the distinction between good and evil, between morally right and morally wrong, society relies and continues to rely on those other distinctions offered by systems which it regards as authoritative in matters concerning children's welfare. Psychoanalysts, for example, may direct the search towards the experiences of the child and its parents during the formative years of life. Political activists, such as feminists and anti-racists, may look to the power relationships that existed at the time within the family and/or the broader social environment. Economists may investigate correlations between income and property of families and the different forms of parenting behaviour. Judges may refer to the weight of the evidence which favours one side rather than another. Cultural relativists may seek the answers in differences in child-rearing customs and traditions. Geneticists may look for family predispositions. Sociologists may seek the answers in social conditions. Moral campaigners may, of course, reformulate all or any of these methods of obtaining the right answer in terms of good or bad for children, but the problem remains that within the social world, outside the moral discourse what counts is not moral formulations, but social communications – the communications of social systems. These are matters which I shall take up in the final chapter.

SOCIETY REVISITED

Autopoietic or self-referential systems

Let me finally in this chapter summarize the notion of society that has been alluded to in the past pages and which provides the framework for the remaining chapters of this book. It derives from the work of the social theorist Niklas Luhmann.

- Like Luhmann, I have argued that to analyse society as if it consisted of people is no longer a useful sociological exercise, given the conditions of modern society. Although people are necessary for society's existence and society is necessary for people's existence, we need to make a clear distinction between people (or conscious systems) and society (social systems). The defining feature of society and what distinguishes it from people, therefore, is communications. This includes all statements, theories, predictions, explanations, results, reports, decisions recommendations, etc. – in fact everything that can be communicated by words, gestures and actions and understood as having meaning. People or conscious systems, on the other hand, may include thoughts, beliefs, ideas, streams of consciousness, conscience and attitudes which exist and remain in an uncommunicated state. Where consciousness is communicated, whether by words, gestures or actions, these communications and the meanings attributed to them will depend upon their interpretations within social systems.

- These differences between social systems reflect the principal organization of modern society into different functions. Each of them operates independently of the particular people who are necessary for producing the communications on which they depend for their distinctive identity. Each of them is closed to its external world in the sense that information from that world cannot penetrate the system in a direct manner. Before it can be recognized by the system, it has to be reproduced in the system's own terms. Only then can it enter the system's programme. These systems are dependent upon other such systems producing and continuing to produce statements, decisions, theories, results or projects within their own spheres. No one of them, however, would be able to replace the knowledge-creating and interpretive functions of other systems. Only law, for example, may decide what is lawful,[6] politics what is national or international policy, science what is factual, religion what is sacred, and economics what constitutes property, and so on. For Luhmann, the term 'social autopoiesis' refers to systems continually referring back to themselves for authority and not to any external source. The term also carries the additional connotation of reproduction through the system's own elements. Anything that is recognized by the system is seen either as part of the system or, alternatively, as existing in that system's environment, that is, external to the system itself.
- At different times in society's history, different systems have come to be seen as privileged in the production of authoritative accounts of social events, which we can call 'authority discourses'. When society was organized hierarchically, religion tended to be treated as the sole or dominant authority discourse. In modern society, with its fragmentation into functionally differentiated systems, the sites of such authority discourses are to be found within the operations of several different systems. These 'authority discourses' may operate in ways which provide society with the prospect of certainty about the past, the present and the future and so come to be relied upon for those decisions which are seen as requiring the impression of finality and authority.

- For both society and its social systems, complexity can be understood in the terms of what is *not accessible* to it. For each system, the existence of complexity makes the system's statements about matters beyond the boundaries of its knowledge dependent upon the operations of other systems, which are not knowable by the system except on its own particular terms. This unknown may be expressed by the term 'contingency', 'the fact that the possibilities of further experience and action indicated in the horizon of actual experience are just that – possibilities – and might turn out differently than expected' that is, that the indications 'might be deceptive' (Luhmann, 1990c, Chapter 2). For each of society's systems, complexity is represented, therefore, by what is not available to that system's particular way of understanding the world. The assurances given by the system are then always contingent upon complexity over which it has no control and no understanding.
- Whatever is accessible to society through its systems of knowledge, is necessarily a reduction of complexity. Through reconstituting elements in its environment – external complexity (or raw data) which has no meaning for the system – into internal complexity, that is into elements which do make sense within the system, which are understandable on the system's terms – the system is able to evolve and reproduce itself. Law, for example, deals with what it perceives as social conflicts by reproducing them in strictly legal terms, according to the concepts existing in legal programmes. It may then apply its own operations to these problems and produce decisions which determine between lawful and unlawful conduct.

For those readers interested in reading more about the theory, a list of writings by Luhmann and other theorists who have developed and applied the idea of closed systems is set out in the references and further reading to this chapter.

EXPLORATIONS

My task in the remainder of this book, I hasten to make clear, does not take the form of a quest for the holy grail of sociology, that elusive, definitive model of society, for as I have explained, society is whatever it is possible to communicate as being society. At one level my purpose is to describe how moral campaigns which claim to know the way to create a better world for children depend for their success upon the construction and dissemination of versions of society and of the social world which recognize only a small part of what is 'known' to sociological observers. In these chapters society no longer consists of a collection of people, and issues are not reduced to a conflict between two (or more) competing belief systems. Instead, I have in each of the chapters taken a specific issue relating to children and their well-being and explored the possibilities that emerge when one observes events as taking place in a world of functionally differentiated systems rather than in less complex moral (or ideological) constructions of society. Several of the chapter begin with a short introduction introducing the reader to any unfamiliar terminology and theoretical concepts that provide a framework for the subsequent exploration.

The results of these explorations may appear uncompromising in their refusal to revert to those certainties, those reassuring territories that are occupied by moral campaigns for children's rights, interests and welfare. They deliberately avoid the firm ground where knowledge is knowledge, data is data and where what is good or bad for children can be ascertained through knowledge, facts and data and then transformed into programmes for changing a child's life, a nation's treatment of children, or the plight of children throughout the world. From the perspective of these explorations there simply is no firm ground; there are no certainties and no reassurances. The conclusions of each chapter may not answer the questions that readers who seek a better world for children want answered, or solve the problems that they want solved. They may, however, take the failures and disappointed expectations of the reader and reconstruct them not as a spur to renewed efforts to find the right answers, but as the starting point for new conceptualizations of problems.

NOTES

1   The generally accepted forms of child abuse are 'physical abuse', 'sexual abuse' and 'ritual abuse', with 'psychological' or 'emotional abuse' as possible additions, although they suffer from problems of definition.
2   A moral philosopher may take an existing set of principles such as Christian ethics or rights for children and 'analyse this set's moral tenets'. But:

More usually the moral philosopher will investigate a moral theory itself investigated and modified by other philosophers. They have either believed it to be a better account than any previous account or than any pre-philosophical doctrine of 'what we all really believe' or have advocated it as an improved guide to practical action.

(Flew, 1979, p. 113)

3 Much of the early writings of Michel Foucault describe how these disciplinary complexes are constructed and reinforced.
4 This does not rule out the possibility that in particular situations or particular times the authority of one or other of the systems may prevail against that of another or others.
5 For a discussion of the danger/risk distinction, see Niklas Luhmann, 1993, Chapter 1, also Ulrich Beck, 1992.
6 Politics, in the form of government, may of course determine the kind of events to which lawful/unlawful determinations should be applied, but cannot itself interpret its own legislation by applying it to particular cases. Only the legal system may take on this role.

Chapter 2

Child abuse and the regulation of male power

INTRODUCTION

Forms and distinctions

The recent preoccupation of the press and news media with child abuse, with the daily discovery of new victims and the unmasking of new villains, has been accompanied at the level of academic inquiry by the publication of huge stacks of books, reports, scientific papers and journal articles all devoted to the subject. Research into symptoms and causes, developing detection techniques, the evaluation of therapeutic treatments, the monitoring of effects, both long-term and short-term, the creation of legal remedies procedures, practices and punishments are forever being published, discussed, criticized, modified. My analysis of the issue of child abuse in this chapter, is not, however, in order to simply add to this mountain of academic papers but rather to offer some reflections upon the nature of anti-child abuse campaigns and to assess the likelihood of their succeeding in their task of controlling abusive behaviour.

Let us start with some preliminary thoughts about the relationship between 'abuse' and 'morality'. It is clear from the start that there is a moral judgment implicit in the word 'abuse'. Abuse is by definition an evil, a wrong, to be prevented and, wherever possible, eliminated. For the purposes of moral condemnation any refinement of the word abuse is redundant. One does not usually talk of 'wicked abuse' or 'evil abuse'. Yet in itself, the term 'abuse' tells us nothing whatsoever about the way that certain kinds of behaviour come to be defined as abusive (and, therefore, immoral) within society at any one time. In the same way the labels 'wicked' and 'evil', in today's society no longer explain adequately the causes of the abuse, as we have seen in the account of the aftermath of the James Bulger murder trial (Chapter 3). Social understanding demands that the causes of social events be found within society itself and not attributed to external forces, whether the devil or the stars.

One can find some general assistance in understanding the ways in which events are defined and causes attributed in George Spencer Brown's theory of distinctions. Niklas Luhmann's writings refer frequently to Spencer Brown's work, *Laws of Form* (1969) as offering an account of the way in which meaning is generated and systems of communication evolve. For Luhmann and Brown any initial statement indicating a difference constitutes a distinction in that it creates a way of perceiving, interpreting and understanding. From that moment onwards future events may be understood in terms of that distinction. The drawing of this first distinction necessarily involves the reduction of complexity, but, as we have seen in Chapter 1, such reductionism is inevitable if events are to have meaning within society and if social knowledge and expectations about the nature of society and people's behaviour in it are to exist within the various systems which are seen as authoritative. In any process of social policy making reducing complexity through the drawing of a distinction is, therefore, a first necessary step in defining an area of concern and formulating strategies for its regulation and control. The very fact that the distinction has been made offers the opportunity for the drawing of further distinctions and these distinctions, to yet more distinctions and the construction of whole bodies of knowledge.

Men and women

The initial man/woman distinction which has proved so important for social organization, for example, presents the opportunity for explanations to be formulated on the basis of gender differences. This in turn makes possible a distinction between explanations that rely on gender difference, and other explanations. Selecting the first side of the distinction, gender difference explanations, will have the effect of reducing complexity to an application of notions of difference between men and women, between the male and the female, and to explanations contrasting the biological nature or social characteristics of men with those of women.

Abuse and harm

The theory of distinctions may also be helpful in identifying the construction of the differences between what comes to be seen as abuse and what does not. Where child abuse is concerned, a common response to a public survey asking what kinds of harm to children are classified as 'abuse' might well be that when abuse occurs it is so obviously abuse that questions of this sort are pointless. Yet what is 'obvious' to all or most people is probably itself based on the distinction between 'obvious' harms – usually a person or people causing physical injury to a child or exploiting children sexually or for profit – on the one hand, and other, more subtle forms of harm to children, such as educational deprivation, long-term damage from pollution, or commercial exploitation through advertising, which, because they are not 'obvious' are not regarded as 'abuse'. Consequently, unless these 'unobvious' forms of abuse provoke a public furore, as where they are seen as being the cause of some outrageous act, as was the fate of 'video nasties' after the Bulger murder trial, there is no pressing obligation upon governments to intervene to regulate or prevent them, or to treat them as an imminent threat to the health and safety of the child, requiring, if necessary, immediate measures designed to rescue children and bring those responsible to justice or treatment. In order to separate the two concepts, there would be some justification in the suggestion that 'abuse' in relation to children tends to be distinguished from those harms which are not seen as abusive, by the existence of an identifiable perpetrator (whether or not the actual identity of the perpetrator is known) and of direct face-to-face contact between perpetrator and victim.

For those who would wish to classify harms to children according to some scale measuring the degree of severity of the damage caused, and so take regulatory steps to prevent the most serious blights to children's lives, there are a number of problems in using the obvious abuse/non-obvious abuse and abusive harm/non-abusive harm distinctions as a guide to action. In the first place, if by harm we mean 'detriment to well-being' both present and future, then it is by no means clear that 'obvious abuse' is more harmful than the long-term effects of emotional and psychological pressures applied to children (Archard, 1993), or of pollution or educational deprivation. Placing a child in a situation where he or she is caught in the middle of a continuing conflict between parents, for example, may well in the long term be more detrimental to that child's future than being bruised or even suffering a broken bone through acts of physical abuse. Second, physical (or even sexual) damage to children may not be as uncontroversial or obviously abusive as it might appear. Third, part or most of the damage may be the result of reactions to the initial harm rather than the harm itself and this secondary harm may be more likely to occur where those harms are classified as abuse. Finally, what constitutes abuse for any social group will depend upon cultural norms or accepted practices. Does a parent hitting a child constitute abuse or lawful disciplining? 'Today's abuse includes much that was yesterday's punishment' (Gordon, 1988, p. 177). Is ritual facial scarring or circumcision abusive when not to be scarred or circumcised would mean that the child would be treated as an outcast by its community? Is causing minor physical injury to children in, for example, punishment for misbehaviour, considered abusive only because it does not conform to prevailing Western child rearing practices?

Clearly there are some kinds of physical damage which would be interpreted as detrimental to the child, wherever or whenever they occurred, but these would probably only include such extreme cases as killing or deliberately maiming children. Any attempt to set out universal guidance as to what constitutes and what does not constitute child abuse which goes beyond such blatant harms is likely to run into cultural barriers. The philosopher, David Archard, in his book, *Children, Rights and Childhood* (1993), for example, proposes 'a commitment to human equality' as a fundamental value which may help to avoid such relativism, but even he then has to admit that there are 'difficult questions' when it comes to applying this principle to 'cultural differences within one and the same society' (p. 152) to say nothing of the problems in tackling these differences on an international scale (see Chapter 7).

This problematic labelling of certain kinds of behaviour as 'abuse' and others as, say, infringements of advertising regulations, the creation of health hazards, or substandard teaching, marks a distinction not between what can be effectively controlled and what cannot, but between what is a matter for moral judgment and what is not. Child sexual and physical abuse, which is the subject of this chapter, clearly is seen as a moral issue and the identification of those responsible and of the causes of abuse which result from the abuse/non-abuse distinction bring into play further distinctions which refer back to the original moral judgment. These searches for perpetrators, victims and causes, therefore, also bring moral judgments into play.

Within any system of morality, beliefs and personal values are important in determining who or what is considered good or bad, moral or immoral at any one time. These beliefs and values may come from many different sources, including religion, political and other ideologies and collective or personal experiences. How and why particular ideas arise as to what kinds of people or what kinds of behaviour are good or bad for children at any one time is a matter for historical observation. It is not our concern here. The focus of this chapter is rather the emergence of one particular moral account of child abuse perpetrators and victims, based on the male/female distinction, and the causes attributed to the abusers. My purpose in writing it is not to take issue directly with this account, but rather to account for the considerable difficulties in translating into social action programmes based on such moral agendas. Where children's welfare is concerned, the failure to apply the moral principles implicit in such agendas to social decision making are usually treated as wholly detrimental to society's future. What I also suggest in this chapter, however, is that when these evaluations of what is good or bad for children and society are subjected to sociological observation, the distinction between a good and bad outcome for both children and society may appear less clear than the promoters of moral campaigns would have us believe. Although their motives of creating a better safer world for children may be morally impeccable, the effects of campaigns to bring about such a desirable state of existence often fail entirely to achieve their objectives or may change society in ways which are very different from those anticipated by the campaigners. In such cases the fact of the fragmentation of authority in modern society may operate in more positive ways than the moral campaigners would recognize. Obstructing the dissemination of 'good' and not recognizing the existence of 'evil' may turn out to be more beneficial for the future of children and society than anyone could have anticipated. Unfortunately, the contingent nature of social events means that there is no way of drawing distinctions which would guarantee in advance what action or inaction will be beneficial to the future of children and society and what will not. This does not, of course, prevent claims based on ideological justifications that such distinctions are not only possible but essential if society is to continue with the belief that it is able improve itself.

Ideologies

Ideology is probably the most frequently used term of all in sociology. It appears on the screen almost every time sociologists place their fingers on computer keyboards. What it means and how it is used varies enormously. At times it becomes confused with such terms as ideas, values, perspectives, but in general it refers to a system of beliefs, often political, which provide people or groups with the motives and justification for their conduct and attitudes. Niklas Luhmann has a particular use for the term 'ideologies'. He describes them as:

> *belief systems* which make it possible for people, either as individuals or collectively, to define societal identity as *a future possibility the realization of which is prevented by certain forces*. This may apply equally to religious, political or scientific schemes of interpretation.
>
> (Luhmann, 1990, pp.127–128, emphasis added)

For Luhmann then the distinguishing features of ideologies are these: first, that they are 'belief systems'; second, that they 'define societal identity' as a future possibility', that is, they look towards some desired future state which may or may not be different from present society; third, the way to this future society is obstructed or threatened by 'certain forces' which the belief system is able to identify. This third element in Luhmann's definition has particular importance for this chapter in that it limits the concept of ideology to those belief systems which make it appear as if there are forces which prevent the realization of the desired future state. Ideology, in Luhmann's hands, becomes, interestingly, a kind of individual or collective paranoia. Ideologies tend to present society not only as something to be 'won over', converted or transformed into something different, but also as containing within it elements which are likely to oppose, or, at least, stand in the way of attempts to change society in the desired direction. Now let us move on to examine the ideology that will form the subject of this chapter and its relation to morality and society as a future possibility.

FEMINIST INSPIRED ANTI-CHILD ABUSE CAMPAIGNS

Feminism is a term which refers to a wide range of theoretical writings centred on women and the female identity as well as to a social movement, which has been particularly influential in changing perceptions of men and women and the relations between them. While some of the theoretical writings, taking as their starting point the distinction between men and women, have been instrumental in formulating new and creative ways of seeing society and the different roles and experiences of women and men in society, by no means all these writings would fit Luhmann's definition of 'ideological'. Feminism as a social (or political) movement clearly falls into this category, depending as it does on 'ideological beliefs making it possible to define a societal identity as a future possibility'. As with many ideologies, the goals of feminist inspired campaigns for social change claim to be based on moral principles. They are concerned, among other things, with justice, with equality, with spiritual improvement and generally with making the world a better place. The most frequently identified force that the social movement sees as preventing or having the potential to prevent the realization of these goals is male power. In much of the literature of what has become known as 'radical feminism' men are seen as possessing a surplus of power – physical, political and economical – which they use to subjugate women and prevent them from achieving such individual goals as self-fulfilment, self-realization, and such social goals as creating a more caring, sensitive, society. Women in this literature tend to be represented as relatively powerless, dominated by men[1] and, often, as the victims of male abuse of power.[2]

This powerful male/powerless female distinction leads us to a further form or classificatory concept which comes to be important in the anti-child abuse campaigns that I shall be examining in this chapter – that of violence. Within moral systems the term violence appears almost always as an evil or a wrong inflicted on victims. People or organizations who wish to act morally do not use violence. Where force is used in a justifiable or morally acceptable way it is rarely, if ever, described by the users as violence, although observers of the use of force may well see it in that way. What is of interest for the purposes of our analysis, however, is not the issue of whether violence can be justified, but rather the way that the notion of violence is used in the hands of many feminist campaigners for social action. Violence here becomes both an unjustifiable evil and an expression of male power.[3] Male violence is defined as a political act, a blatant expression of domination whether it takes the form of rape or physical or sexual assaults in public places or the beating of wives by husbands and children by fathers occurring in the privacy of the home.

Whether men should bear the burden of blame for their violent behaviour or whether this burden should be shared between men and women is clearly an important, if controversial, moral issue which is left unexplored by radical feminists, who begin their inquiries already equipped with the answer to that question. What particularly concerns us here, however, is the fact that feminist moral campaigns tend to link male violence with power in a way that leads to the conclusion either that it is only men who use violence or that only men use violence for the purposes of dominating and subjugating others.

The American feminist writer, Jan Stets, for example, reports that 'men use violence to dominate, control and force women to conform to what they want' and that 'men want to determine how their partners behave, and the way they do this is through violence . . .' (Stets 1988, pp. 109 and 110),[4] while another American feminist, Martha Mahoney, describes the situation in which women find themselves needing: 'legal and social explanations of women's experience that illuminate the issue of violence as part of the issue of power, rather than perpetuating or exacerbating the images that now conceal questions of domination and control' (Mahoney, 1991, p. 5).

To 'illuminate the issue of violence as part of the issue of power may, according to Catherine MacKinnon, be a major problem for women, because: 'In a society of gender inequality, the speech of the powerful impresses its view on the world, concealing the truth of powerlessness under a despairing acquiescence that provides the appearance of consent and makes protest inaudible as well as rare (MacKinnon, 1989, p. 205).

The moral campaigns against child abuse inspired by these ideas take up the notion of male power and its concealment. They present a vision of male dominance, usually expressed through violence or the threat of violence as being the only valid explanation for physical and sexual assaults on children. Alternative explanations operate to conceal this truth. The Australian feminist lawyer, Hilary Astor, maintains all male violence *within the family*, whether or not directed at the children, is in itself harmful to children, because it has grave effects on the child, including, in the short term, 'a high rate of medical problems such as insomnia, diarrhoea, heartache, asthma and also a high rate of behavioural problems, while the long-term effects on the child are behavioural and emotional problems' (Astor, 1991, pp. 16–17).

From within their belief system, these writers observe men's conduct and male power as the obstacle to the realization of a society which would be free of violence and where children would no longer be the victims of oppression and exploitation. They would argue that it is the concealment and failure to recognize this fact which stands in opposition to the realization of a better world for both women and children.

The feminist historian, Linda Gordon, however, points to the limitations of this approach when she considers the case of women who abuse children:

> The role of women as child abusers is important because child abuse is the only form of family violence in which women's assaults are common. Studying child abuse thus affords an unusual opportunity to examine women's anger and violence. Unfortunately, feminist influence in anti-family-violence work has not historically supported such an examination, because of an ideological emphasis on women's peaceableness and a rejection of victim-blaming that have pervaded much of feminist thought.
>
> (Gordon, 1988a, p. 173)

Similarly, White and Farmer, in considering sexually aggressive behaviour by men argue that:

> [A]lthough the feminist assumptions concerning sexual aggression illuminated facets of sexual assault that had previously been ignored (i.e. patriarchal values, the role of power, and dominance motives), exclusive adherence to such assumptions can result in an incomplete understanding of sexual violence.
>
> (White and Farmer, 1992)

Yet many feminist writers and observers of feminist campaigns against child abuse have argued that the interpretation of the causes of physical and sexual abuse on children which stresses male power and men's violence was essential to counter prevailing interpretative frameworks which ignored patriarchy as a factor and emphasized gender-neutral, psychological and social causes (McLoed and Saraga, 1988; Nava, 1988). It is, of course, quite right that these previous accounts of the causes of child abuse should be subjected to critical analysis and that others should be at liberty to offer their own alternative explanations. One would perhaps expect these critics to welcome the same attention from those observers who are doubtful of the cogency of their particular accounts of causality. Often, however, such attention has been treated by anti-child abuse campaigners as 'part of the problem', as a manifestation of that very concealment of power that the campaigners are determined to reveal as blocking the way to progress towards a better society.

There is an additional problem for those radical feminists who seek to save children from what they see as the harms resulting from expressions of 'masculinity', whom I shall from now on refer to as 'anti-child abuse campaigners'. Assuming that these campaigners are right in their identification of the 'forces' which prevent 'the realization of their societal possibilities', how can this recognition be translated into social action? How, in the terms with which we began this book, can the moral principles of the anti-abuse campaigners find expression in those social systems that society sees as authoritative? What forms precisely could the effective control of male violence take?

THE REGULATION OF MALE POWER

If anti-child abuse campaigners were able themselves to take direct action against abusing men, the general objective of their policies would be to reduce the opportunities for violence and ensure that where men were violent, they could expect their losses to far outweigh any gains. Men could, for example, be banned from any contact with the children that they had abused. They could also be severely punished for the abuse by long prison sentences, which, as well as separating the abuser from the victim, could act as a deterrent to other potential abusers. Another strategy might be to regard men who were violent to children as 'sick' and to subject them to forcible treatment. Physical violence or sexual exploitation could be regarded as illnesses or as the results of some disorder which required medical intervention through drugs, aversion therapy or periods of enforced hospitalization, at the end of which, hopefully, the abusive men would learn how to control their behaviour and to recognize the harm it was causing to the child. All these remedies for child abuse have in fact been proposed at one time or another by anti-child abuse campaigners, even if not all of them have been put into practice. Naturally, they are directed exclusively at men, while women who hit, exploit, or fail to protect children against such violence or exploitation tend to be seen as acting not as abusers, but as themselves the victims of patriarchal oppression. It is the men in their lives and, more sociologically, society's aberrant construction of masculinity which is seen as being 'the problem' to be solved, the conduct to be controlled. For women direct action takes the form of providing help and support to resist male domination. According to MacLoed and Saraga, therefore:

> Until and unless it is recognized that child sexual abuse is a gender issue, and a product of the social construction of masculinity, there can be no change, either in individual men or in masculinity, no counter to the view of masculinity.
>
> (MacLoed and Saraga, 1988, p. 52)

This leads to the second category of direct measures designed to control male power. By empowering the victims of oppression the imbalance caused by men's superior physical strength, economic control and aggressiveness may be redressed. Women would be in a better position to protect children, by, for example, removing them from the reach of abusing men. Children too, if empowered, would be more capable of seeking help and of resisting the brute force or economic pressures exerted by men against their interests. According to this method of regulating male power, the task of protective social work would be primarily that of intervening at the request and on the side of women and children to help them to combat male oppression (Dominelli and McLoed, 1989).

In the longer term, however, the only effective regulation of the problem of child abuse would, according to the perspective of these anti-child abuse campaigners, appear to lie in the total transformation of society from its present patriarchal state to one in which women had much more control over their own lives and were thereby able to protect their children against men's oppressive and abusive behaviour. There is a problem here: it is never made clear how precisely this new society would differ from the present one. It is clear in only one respect, which is that women would have much more power and much greater authority over the decision making processes affecting their lives and those of their children than occurs at present (MacKinnon, 1989). Apart from this, it would seem that all the institutions of society, except perhaps the family, would remain very much as they are at present. In so far as regulating child abuse is concerned, the notion of society that these anti-child abuse campaigners draw upon is not so much a utopian vision of Marxian dimensions, but a world where moral campaigns are able to lead directly to action being taken by society's institutions to prevent the harm and, eventually, eliminate the evil that they, the campaigners, have identified.

For autopoietic theory, the difficulty for anti-child abuse campaigners lies not in the moral message that they wish to convey, but in their ideological (or paranoid!) account of society as consisting essentially of a collection of social institutions, each in its way supporting male domination and oppressing women and children, each contributing to the imbalance of power between men and women and to the social construction of masculinity. It is these male-dominated institutions which are seen ideologically as representing the forces opposed to a better society and yet the anti-child abuse campaigners are obliged to rely upon the continuing operations of these institutions to achieve their vision of a better society.

The problem seen in autopoietic terms is by now a familiar one. It consists of finding ways to transform moral statements into social action, given the fragmented nature of authority in modern society and the self-referring nature of the social systems which society has designated as sites of authority. Put in more precise terms, social change has to occur within society and is distinct from changing people's beliefs and attitudes. These beliefs and attitudes may act as precursors or irritants to social change, but they need to be transformed into authoritative knowledge before society will recognize them.[5] Changes within society's systems of authoritative knowledge, however, do not depend on the force of the moral message, but on the system's own internal, self-referential operations, its programmes. There can be no guarantee, therefore, that irritants or perturbations within the system's environment will produce the desired change within the system. Ideological campaigns based on expectations that society and its institutions will be open and amenable to change through direct influence or pressure carry with them a heavy risk of disappointment. With this in mind, let us see how anti-child abuse campaigns have fared in their attempts to gain acceptance for their moral agendas.

ANTI-CHILD ABUSE WITHIN SOCIAL SYSTEMS

The four social systems that I shall discuss here are science, law, politics and economics, as it is the communications of these systems which have proved most authoritative for society in its construction and development of controls and regulations for the detection and diagnosis of, and social responses to, child abuse. The task is to see how the strategies of anti-child abuse campaigns have fared and are likely in future to fare in bringing their moral message into the programmes of these systems.

Science

The authoritative role that science fulfils in modern society, as we have seen (pages 18–19) is that of producing facts on which society can rely, that is, it distinguishes between what is factual for society and what is fictional. Clearly then, if the campaigners' explanatory accounts of child abuse could be shown to be scientifically true, if in other words the cause of the abusing behaviour could be incontrovertibly traced to masculinity, patriarchy and the exercise of male power then   all other social systems, including law and politics would be obliged to take account of this scientific fact and adapt themselves in various ways to its existence.

In order to succeed scientifically the campaigners would have to convince the scientific establishment first, that *all abuse* against children was directly or indirectly the product of men's oppressive conduct, and second, that this conduct was the result of their masculinity, whether the cause of this masculinity was biologically or socially constructed. They would have to discredit, for example, explanations about the contribution of men's own childhood experiences as victims of both physical violence and sexual assaults (White and Farmer, 1992). They would also need to have dismissed as scientifically false accounts of harmful behaviour towards children which looked to stress, drug or alcohol use, or the interpersonal dynamics of the family system as providing a valid explanation for some or all child abuse.[6] These are formidable tasks.

The vast child abuse literature contains many hundreds of research reports, articles and book chapters on many aspects of these controversial issues. Yet not one of these has been able to provide the incontrovertible evidence that would be necessary to establish that one and only one explanation is correct and all others are wrong, or even that, generally, one version is more probably correct than others. Rather it would appear that much depends upon how a particular issue concerning behaviour towards children is formulated and what factors are pre-selected for scientific investigation. Probably the most that can be said is that one particular explanation may appear convincing for some cases, while other kinds of interpretations seem to be better for others. In every instance, however, there is always room for more than one explanatory framework for the same set of events.

The scientific conclusion would have to be, therefore, that it is not possible for science to identify one kind of explanation as definitive or generally the most convincing. Such judgments cannot be scientifically based. They will depend not upon scientific criteria, but upon which explanatory framework appears most compelling to the particular interpreter. Explanations based on the notion of male power are, therefore, no more convincing as science than many other explanations. If they are to be reformulated as science they must take their place among other accounts as possible versions of truth. Nor is there any prospect that further research will provide more certainty as to the real causes of child abuse. The fundamental problem is that the very notion of 'child abuse' covers so many social situations that it is impossible to reduce it to dimensions which can be investigated as if it were a simple physical phenomenon, where all the variables which contributed to its existence could be individually investigated or controlled .

Law

The difficult task for anti-child abuse campaigns directed at changing the law is to push the legal process in one direction and one direction only, that of redressing the harms and injustices produced by male power. This means, in effect, demanding that law rejects all causal explanations for child abuse except those which point to men's behaviour. It requires the law to conceptualize child abuse as the product of male power and female (or child) powerlessness. It is the violent expression of male power which law needs to regulate. At the same time, the law is expected to reject or ignore all other possible explanations, such as those associated with cultural difference or individual pathology, unassociated with gender. Yet, given the scripts law writes for itself (its programmes) and its definition of its own boundaries and environment (see pages 17–19), it has to 'do justice' not just to women and mothers, but to all those different individuals and interest groups which appear in its environment as demanding justice and the resolution of disputes. Failures of the legal system to satisfy these demands are likely to result in legal decisions losing their authority to the detriment of all other social systems which are obliged to rely upon legal certainties for their own operations.

Furthermore, it is according to notions of children's welfare and criminal responsibility that child abuse cases are processed by the law's programmes, and not according to concepts of power and patriarchy. While the legal system may not be able to assess from the application of its own programmes what is or will be good or bad for children, it will usually be able to reproduce within these programmes available scientific (or medical) information concerning, for example, the likely effects of violence on children's well-being and the risks involved in returning children to a violent parent. For matters involving children's welfare the legal decision is a just decision, not merely because it is lawful, but also because it has been made in conformity with the best available 'expert evidence'.[7]

When it comes to decisions about children's welfare, therefore, lawfulness, and so justice, involves something rather different than political or moral philosophical notions of justice. It may also be different from the view of justice taken by anti-child abuse campaigners. Yet the choices available to law in its selections from science communications will not depend on science, but on law. Which evidence is seen as compelling and which expert is recognized as authoritative will, of course, depend upon legal rather than scientific programmes, but this does not solve the problems for the promoters of these campaigns. The space in law that was once available for morality has now been filled by science and so there is no way that campaigners can avoid the difficult task of convincing the courts that their scientific evidence is more compelling and their experts are more convincing than others on where the child's best interests lie.

It might be thought that the lack of scientific certainty over the causes of child abuse and predictions of what course of action will best serve the child's welfare, which we discussed earlier, would leave a space to be filled within law's programmes by moral judgments. For example, the question as to whether a child should continue to have contact with a parent who has behaved in a violent way towards that child cannot be answered satisfactorily through scientific evidence. There may be sound scientific arguments on both sides. Ultimately any judgment, it would seem, will be made by deciding between conflicting beliefs concerning the needs of the child. These beliefs may be traced to different moral positions, which differ in their identification of 'the good' and 'the bad', 'the right' and 'the wrong'. Indeed, a court's decision on whether it is right for a violent father to continue to have contact with his child or whether that father should forfeit any right to see his child may well subsequently come to be observed in moral terms, in which case, whether the decision is seen as morally right as well as legally right will depend, in the absence of any consensual version of morality, upon the particular moral view taken by different observers. Today, however, within the legal system itself, the co-evolution of law with child welfare science has left virtually no space for such moral observations. It is the weight of scientific evidence which is seen as justifying the correctness of the decision, and not morality. This will be the case despite the best efforts of the anti-child abuse campaigners and despite their *ex post facto* criticisms of legal decisions.

One can understand the anger and frustration of critical observers of legal decisions when confronted by male judges who refuse to see relations within families in terms of gender and generation power (e.g. Wells, 1994). Yet the problem, as I have explained, may not lie so much with the prejudices of male judges as with law's task of stabilizing expectations about children and their well-being. The controversial nature of a morality based on resistance to patriarchy and male violence is unlikely to prove attractive to a legal system even if it were to take the unlikely step of abandoning its reliance on scientific (or medical) expertise. For this to change, there would first have to be changes in the law's perception of the kind of authority likely to stabilize society's expectations concerning children and their well-being. It would not be sufficient merely to substitute women judges for male judges. There would also need to be changes in law's selection of information on what might be good or bad for children. Either the science that law reformulated in its programmes and operations would have to recognize the fact of male domination as the principal cause of harm to children or the coupling of law and child welfare science would have to give way to other combinations, such as politics-within-law or morality-within-law. Neither of these events seem likely.

It might be supposed that anti-child abuse campaigners might prove more successful in criminal prosecutions against the alleged perpetrators of abuse, for here the welfare of the child and thus scientific accounts of children's interests, take a secondary place to such issues of public policy as deterrence of and retribution for socially harmful acts. Here again, however, the moral objectives of these campaigns run up against the problem of their reformulation within law. The goal of bringing male abusers of power to account, so that they can be punished or ordered by the courts to subject themselves to treatment or retraining is often thwarted by legal rules of evidence and procedure which seek to protect 'the accused' against wrongful conviction, or by organizational guidances which, for reasons of economy and efficiency, rule out prosecutions in the absence of sufficiently compelling evidence. In Britain, for example, prosecutions of alleged sex abusers of very young children are rarely undertaken in the absence of forensic evidence or a confession by the abuser. The ordeal for a young child of giving evidence combined with a strong probability of such evidence being rejected by a jury as unreliable are seen as good reasons for not prosecuting, regardless of the harm caused to the child or strong beliefs in the guilt of the suspect. Even where older children are concerned, prosecutors' subjective assessments of the child's likely performance as a witness play a significant part in determining whether the case will go ahead.[8] Attempts to overcome the obstacles to prosecution through such techniques as live video links and video recordings of children's evidence have gone some way towards increasing the likelihood of prosecution and conviction, but anti-child abuse campaigns can only go a certain distance in this direction before they run up against the the law's procedural demands aimed at minimizing the risks of wrongful convictions.

The introduction in some American states of specialist domestic violence courts where the judges and court staff are almost all women, may give anti-child abuse campaigners some cause for optimism. Here, it seems the moral value of protecting women against violent men is raised above all others. These courts are able to convey the message that, contrary to some cultural beliefs, beating women is wrong. They may order men to stay away from the women they have assaulted and punish disobedience of court injunctions with imprisonment. They may order men who have been habitually violent to attend treatment programmes to improve their behavioural control and their attitude towards women and punish them for their non-cooperation. Yet any attempt to introduce similar courts for child abuse would be likely to encounter considerable difficulties. Would they apply, for example, only to men or would mothers who abused their children be equally liable to prosecution and punishment? Would mothers who protected their male child-abusing partner by not reporting the abuse or refusing to give evidence also risk punishment? Would fathers be gaoled for continuing to see their children after a court injunction, even where the mother collaborated in the arrangement? Clearly, success would be likely only in those cases where the man only had abused the child and the woman had decided to separate permanently from him and to keep him away from the children. Only in such situations would it be possible for the law to distinguish between the man and the woman as separate legal entities rather than regarding them both as 'parents' or 'caretakers' jointly responsible for ensuring the children's welfare. The problems would, of course, be even greater in cases of child sexual abuse, where the law's insistence on sufficient proof would be likely to result in long, protracted cases to establish 'the facts' before any firm action could be taken.

Politics

Perhaps moral campaigns to protect children from abuse can expect more success in the political sphere, where ideologies rather than notions of truth or legality compete to promote their particular society and to overcome those forces which prevent its realization. Yet before jumping to any optimistic conclusions, one needs to examine the operations of the political system in those situations where the source of its authority is 'the will of the people', meaning the majority (howsoever defined) of the electorate. Political communications, intended for external consumption, are directed at those who have the capacity to return the present government to power or to replace it. Within the publicly contested debates between government and opposition, each side remains convinced as to the correctness of its position, the validity of its vision and the falseness or absurdity of the claims of the opposing party. From the outset and throughout the debate government and opposition publicly agree only to the proposition that no agreement between them on matters of political significance can be or should be possible.

The truths of the one are reconstituted as falsehoods within the communications of the other. This is not to say that these truths (and falsehoods) will not change over time. Political parties have even been known historically to exchange truths and falsehoods, so that the truths of one party become its falsehoods when, at some later time, they are adopted as truths by the other party. But in politics, unlike science, the inspiration for changes of position is rarely the emergence of new evidence on the subject matter of the debate and nothing more. It is much more likely to be changes in the internal programme of the political system itself making a change of policy expedient or necessary for the purposes of winning or retaining power.

In broad terms the problems that anti-child abuse campaigns are likely to encounter within politics will relate to the mismatch between their moral vision of an abuse-free society and those political programmes which are designed for the primary purpose of winning power and support for that power. This does not mean that only those policies expected to attract popular support are politically acceptable, but rather that unpopularity is not a state to be tolerated in the long term. Policies must be seen within the political system as leading in the short or long term (and preferably both) to outcomes that will attract popular support.

In similar terms this intolerance of unpopularity does not in itself necessarily disqualify from government or opposition policy the agendas of moral campaigners. Both a government with the security of a large majority and an opposition party which has no possibility of becoming the majority party may well look to moral principles for policy guidance. What it does mean, however, is that for any party that takes seriously its prospects of gaining or holding onto power, the formulation of moral values as party policy cannot take place independently of the ultimate need to win or retain the confidence of the electorate in its ability to maintain order and to steer the country (or state) to better times. It may very well, for example, find attractive the principle that violence should be discouraged and controlled, but it is likely to find rather less attractive the notion that what needs to be changed through its policies is masculinity or the male self-image, which lies behind expressions of violence. Moreover, where competing political parties rely upon such slogans as 'the party of the family' or 'the upholders of family values' there is likely to be resistance within politics to moral communications which see the breaking up of families as preferable to keeping them together, even where the outcomes for some of the individuals who make up these families would probably be improved by not staying within the family unit.

For anti-child abuse campaigners to succeed in the political sphere in obtaining support for policies based on their particular version of child abuse and its causality, they would need to formulate the issue as one which has a clear message for politics. In other words, they would need to convince either government or opposition that there are political rewards, whether long or short term, to be gained by taking sides in a debate which identifies men, and only men, as the cause of harm to children.

One difficulty for these campaigners is that political parties wishing to obtain or retain power will tend to select those items from the group's proposals which they believe will gain popular appeal, and ignore the rest.[9] The response of government and opposition in Britain, for example, to campaigns designed to 'put violence against women on the political agenda' was an acceptance of the fact of domestic violence, but a clear rejection of the feminist message that the sole or principal cause of that violence is the power differential between men and women. In 1975 in the United Kingdom, for example, the Select Committee on Violence in Marriage came to what is a disappointing conclusion for radical feminists by stating that there was

> no evidence that the husband alone is responsible for his violence. The behaviour of the wife is relevant. So, too, is the family's environment, their housing and employment conditions, their physical and mental health, their sexual relationship and many other factors.
>
> (Select Committee on Violence in Marriage, p. VIII)

Reconstructed within politics, the phenomenon of domestic violence tended to become a problem like those of crime control, housing, education, alcohol consumption and child protection, leaving both government and opposition free to impose the particular account of causality that accorded with the political ideology they wished to convey to the electorate. In a similar manner, physical violence against and sexual exploitation of children within the family risk being formulated within politics as problems of efficiency and professional judgment for social workers (see Chapter 6). Policy programmes promising well organized, sensitive but effective child protection agencies are probably more likely to gain popular support than a commitment to make fathers the target of interventionist child protecting strategies. At least the former are not likely to upset or alienate a significant number of voters.[10] This is not to suggest that anti-child abuse campaigners who try to persuade governments to accept their way of seeing things will never experience any success. Recent events in New Zealand belie such a suggestion. There, the government recently passed a law stating that in cases of divorce and separation coming before the courts where domestic violence is proved, there shall be no order for custody or unsupervised access to the violent party, unless the court is satisfied that the child would be safe.[11] My purpose here is rather to point out the obstacles in translating the campaigners' moral agenda into political terms.

The other difficulty, which even the New Zealand legislation is hardly likely to overcome, affects all those, whether they be moral campaigners or political parties, who put their faith in politics' capacity to improve society simply by its own actions. Such visions tend seriously to overestimate what can be achieved through political action. In practice, all that the political system is able to do is, first, to pass laws and second, to spend money without being accountable for any losses. Yet the problems for those who want to guarantee the success of a radical feminist campaign against child abuse does not end with the passing of laws. Seen from an autopoietic systems perspective, neither politics nor legislative acts have the ability to control society. New laws may enter the environments of other systems as authoritative political communications, but inevitably these systems construe them in ways that make sense to that system alone. Faced with having to implement the new law, the New Zealand legal system is likely to insist upon its rules of evidence and procedure being followed in determining whether alleged acts of violence are proved or not. It will also have to consider the welfare of the child and the likelihood of the violence continuing. This will leave the way open for child welfare experts to present evidence in court which will not necessarily conform with feminist accounts of the causality of domestic violence. Economically, this assumption against contact between father and children may have unfortunate financial consequences. It may be used as a bargaining counter in the negotiations for financial settlements following divorce or separation; it may involve the legal aid fund or the parent(s) in the funding of long complicated legal battles to decide whether or not the assumption should be followed in particular cases and, where it is upheld, it may have adverse effects on the willingness of fathers to pay for their children's upkeep. Finally, the new law will enter the environment of the family system as a perturbation to existing emotional relationships. Some children, particularly older ones, may well not accept the no-contact rule and continue to see their absent fathers in spite of court rulings to the contrary. Others may refuse to maintain contact in defiance of a court order that the assumption should not apply. Success in any one system, therefore, is no guarantee that all the communications which constitute society will change in the direction predicated by communications emerging from that system.

Economics

The economic system is concerned with money and property and within that system's programmes people – men, women and children – appear as assets, investments, liabilities, consumers, owners, buyers, sellers, etc. Economics has no way of distinguishing gender and age differences except in these terms. Other systems appear in economics also in terms of the costs and benefits of their programmes and the communications of these systems are reformulated and evaluated according to their impact on such economic programmes as stock markets, profit–loss accounts, trade balances, and currency exchange levels. While political power authorizes governments to spend money without the need to account for losses or to make profits, economics may in its turn provide authority for political action, particularly where, as in today's world, national governments are seen as the managers of their country's economy and success or failure in elections may depend to a considerable degree upon whether the government is seen as having carried out its management tasks well or badly. This coupling of politics and economics, of course, has important repercussions for the outcome of moral campaigns and the reconstitution of their demands within government or opposition programmes but, once again, not in ways that are foreseeable from any moral evaluation of the principles guiding these campaigns. In other words, success or failure in such campaigns does not depend upon morality or appeals to moral principles, but on other factors, to which moral programmes are blind.

To put the matter at its bluntest, those moral agendas which are probably going to cost a government large sums of money in, for example, setting up agencies to enforce the law or paying out benefits to victims are less likely to receive support than those which require very little expenditure. The same is true where it can be anticipated that the principle-based policy is likely to make people or organizations less productive, disrupt ongoing work patterns or result in substantial payments from the public purse.

If economic knowledge provides any authority for anti-child abuse campaigns, it will probably do so by drawing attention to the losses to be expected from not taking action rather than the gains to be anticipated from government or other intervention programmes. As long as scientific knowledge, for example, is available to point to the dysfunctional effects of violence upon families and, in particular, the children of those families, there is some possibility of such information being translated into economic terms with negative outcomes being projected onto future generations, the so-called 'cycle of deprivation'. An economic analysis might recognize that only by intervention, whether through providing refuges for mothers and children, or legal measures to exclude the violent man from the home, may the cycle be broken and future losses avoided or reduced.

A more common situation is for economic programmes to operate as a damper upon the enthusiasm of anti-child abuse campaigns by emphasizing the cost involved in protecting children in ways that conform with the campaigners belief that it is the misuse of power by men that is responsible for the abuse of children. Such negative assessments from economics are even more likely in a society which tends to values men's uninterrupted productive labour above that of women, whose careers are likely to be interrupted by childbirth and child rearing. As long as this situation prevails, any authority to be derived from economic analysis may well be inclined to support the prevention of undue disruption in men's lives rather than protecting women and children against violent men.

There is, however, no guarantee that this situation will not alter as technological developments and demographic factors are translated into economic programmes. A devaluing of childbirth, for example, could lead to many more women pursuing uninterrupted careers and in turn this might change the evaluation of measures to deal with violent men. These are complex and speculative issues and as such tend to be invisible to anti-child abuse campaigners where an ideological commitment to rescuing children and the prevention of imminent harm tends to limit the scope of their perspective to the possibilities for immediate interventionist action.

Campaigns against male violence against and sex abuse of children, therefore, rarely refer to these economic factors or propose ways of regulating them, but tend to concentrate on the interpersonal and the psychological. This is not surprising, since the ideological programme on which such campaigns are founded is not an economic programme and as such has nothing to say about the existing economic order, except that men, rather than women, dominate; or about the way that any new economic order should be established, except to say that this inequality should be redressed and this unjust situation should be rectified.

THE CERTAINTY OF UNCERTAINTY

Moral campaigns depend for their energy and impulsion upon certainty in the rightness of their cause. In a society which has embraced uncertainty as the only guide to the future, it is, therefore, not altogether surprising that the efforts of moral campaigners to convert moral convictions into social achievements should encounter so much resistance. If we knew for certain the nature of future disasters, we would all join together in trying to avoid them. Yet all we really know about the future is that it will not be like the past or like the present, and no more than that. The problem for the radical feminist anti-child abuse campaigns, as for all other moral crusades, is that, in order for its message to be communicable, it has to assume that success would change the social world only in conformity with its moral agenda. In the absence of some vision of a post-patriarchal world, it has to assume that the structures and programmes of existing social organizations will remain intact. Yet we all know that the very fact that women would in this future world be either equal or dominant participants in these organizations would itself be the effect of other societal changes, and that they will themselves produce the conditions for other changes, although it is impossible to predict what these changes will have been or might be.

Faced with the particular social problem of child abuse, nothing is more certain than our uncertainty, not only concerning what action today will be good or bad for children tomorrow, but also in relation to the very concept of child abuse. Linda Gordon tells us that '[T]oday's abuse includes much that was yesterday's punishment' (1988, p. 177). It is also true that tomorrow's forms of child abuse will be different from today's, and whatever the forms they take, the causes and effects attributed to them will also be different from those of today's radical feminist campaigners or the alternatives to their attributions. It would be unreasonable to expect such an analysis to dampen the enthusiasm of anti-child abuse campaigners. On the contrary, it would be more reasonable to expect them to redouble their efforts in the face of uncertainty, like religious sects when their prophesies of armageddon fail to materialize.[12]

For an observer of social systems, the real problem for these campaigners, or in Luhmann's terms, the forces that prevent the realization of their societal identity as a future possibility, is not, as they believe and would have us believe, 'men' and the 'patriarchy', but a society which can do nothing with moral certainties except convert them through its social systems into communications which appear certain, but will always, because of their contingent nature, contain within them an element of uncertainty. Whether we believe this element of uncertainty to be advantageous or disadvantageous for society's future, and indeed the future of society's children, is a matter of conviction. Those who are undecided might, however, remind themselves, before they leap onto the wagon of certainty, that today's certainties often prove to be tomorrow's heresies and today's heresies, tomorrow's certainties.

NOTES

1 See Gordon, 1988; MacKinnon, 1989; Pahl, 1985; Radford and Russell, 1992; Smart, 1989; Wolf, 1993.
2 See, for example, Blackburn and Tooze, 1994; Pahl, 1985; MacLoed and Saraga 1988; Kelly, 1988; Fischer et al., 1993; Russell, 1984; Bayer and Conners, 1988. This does not mean to say that this gender classification cannot be combined with others, such as class or race, to produce quite complex and sophisticated analyses of power combining two or more different codings.
3 See Stets, 1988; MacKinnon, 1989; Kirsta, 1994; Gordon, 1988(a and b); Herman, 1993; Astor, 1991; Hanmer et al., 1989; Pahl, 1985.
4 It needs to be said that not all feminist writers would see social relations in such stark binary terms. Carol Smart, for instance, writes: 'Any argument that starts with ceding priority to the binary division of male/female or masculine/feminine walks into the trap of demoting other forms of differentiation, particularly differences within these binary opposites' (Smart, 1992, p. 34).
5 See pages 24–26.
6 See Pahl, 1985; Fischer, 1993.
7 'The opinion of scientific men upon proven facts may be given by men of science within their own science.' Lord Mansfield in the case of Foulkes v. Chadd 3, Doug. (1782). See also Michael King and Christine Piper, 1995; Michael King and Judith Trowell, 1992; Brian Wynne, 1989.
8 See Wattam (1992) for a report of the factors taken into account in prosecutors' assessments of children's reliability and of the effects of these assessments on decisions (p. 58).
9 Some social theorists have described this process in terms of the reconstruction of social problems (Spector and Kitsuse, 1977; Manning, 1985), but such descriptions appear to be based upon the

supposition that raw or unreconstructed social problems are able to exist. This supposition would be rejected by autopoietic theory.
10 Legislation which appears to discriminate in favour of one sex and against another, such as the Child Support Act, is always likely to be controversial and politically risky.
11 Domestic Violence Act, 1995 which became effective on 1st July 1996.
12 See Leon Festinger, 1964.

Chapter 3

Juridification in the protection of the Scottish child

THE PARADOXICAL NATURE OF SOCIAL SYSTEMS

This chapter looks at the problems posed for the objective of protecting children by the paradoxical nature of those systems that society expects to be responsible for such protection – the paradox of their own existence. What this refers to is not the logician's idea of a paradox, meaning a proposition that appears to contain its own negation – such as the sentence 'This statement is false' – nor is it statements that simply contradict one another. The concept of social systems' paradox lies rather in the manner in which these systems are constituted. As I explained in the first chapter, for the purposes of our analysis social systems are seen as consisting of groupings of knowledge and understanding. As such, the version of their environment (the world, society, or any part of them) that they are capable of recognizing is limited by their own coding, such as lawful/unlawful, government/opposition, scientifically true/scientifically false and profit/loss, pass/fail, sacred/profane, etc. Since there can be no direct access to the totality of social reality (complexity) except through that system's coding, each system in effect creates its own reality. The only way that social systems are able to come into existence and, once created, maintain their identity as separate systems, is by distinguishing themselves from the general environment in which they exist, determining what represents the system and what is the environment for that system. Since the system's and the environment's existence both depend upon the system's initial coding, the only way that it is able to achieve this distinction is through its own operations, so that the system/environment distinction itself becomes a product of those operations. Religion, for example, operates on the basis that only religious operations are able to determine what specifically constitutes religious belief and practice, scientific operations what constitutes truth, legal operations what constitutes justice, political operations what constitutes politics, and so on, with each system referring back to itself in order to decide what it is and where it begins and ends. Each system is then the authority for its own knowledge and the validity of its communications.

This paradox of self-observation becomes particularly problematic for contemporary society when its occurs in society's social function systems. Take, for example, science, which, since the Enlightenment, has been given the task of determining 'truth' for society. The code which governs its internal operations and by which science constructs the external environment, is that of 'true/false' or 'true/not true'. Science, therefore, distinguishes itself from its environment by the specificity and uniqueness of its identity, yet since any communication is subjected by science to science's coding (or selectivity), how can science be sure that its claim to be capable of distinguishing truth from falsehood is in fact 'true'? The claim rests entirely on science's construction of an environment in which it itself appears capable of making such judgments of truth and falsehood.

The legal system, which claims to operate on the basis of just/unjust, in a similar manner finds itself confronting a paradoxical situation in which law poses the problem of its own justice or, at least, applies that distinction to its own observations of external reality.[1] Law's authority, based on its ability to 'do justice', is itself subject to the legal system's coding of legal/illegal, lawful/unlawful. Justice may, therefore, be either lawful or unlawful, with the resultant paradoxes of 'lawfully unjust', as in disobedience of an unjust law or 'unlawfully just', when a person takes the law into his own hands. Within the environment constructed by law the paradox of justice/injustice is resolvable only by transforming it into the distinction, lawful/unlawful – a distinction that may be made by law and law alone.[2]

Paradoxes represent a problem, not necessarily for the system which operates on the basis of the paradox, but for the observer of the system who is able to see both the system and its environment from a different perspective from that of the system. Politics, for example, may well be able to distinguish between justice and legality, at least in certain cases, and declare that a law is unjust. The paradox of the system's identity may become a problem for the system in those situations where the observations of other systems become irritants for the system. This may happen where the perceived injustices of the legal system undermine its communications to the extent that there are doubts over the certainty of its lawful/unlawful decisions. In a similar manner the authority of scientific discoveries may be diminished by doubts over their validity as representing absolute truth. The social and psychological sciences are particularly vulnerable to this kind of disturbance to their self-assurance.

In order to maintain their distinct identity (and thus their authority), these systems from time to time may need transformation from paradoxes into distinctions. For law this process of 'deparadoxification' – this substitution of distinctions so as to conceal the fact that it is law, through its own operations and reconstruction of the external world, which is deciding the meaning for society of justice and injustice, and not some supreme authority – is a particularly rich source of creativity, obliging law to find ever more inventive ways of masking the appearance of paradoxes. Take for example what appears to an external observer to be an unjust or wrongful criminal conviction. Within law this injustice gives rise to the paradox of lawful but unjust. Law's only way of dealing with injustice is to declare the decision lawful or unlawful. In other words, the legal system is unable to recognize an unjust decision as an injustice as long as it remains a 'lawful' decision. In order to deparadoxify the paradox of lawfully unjust, the legal system must through its operations reconstitute the situation in ways which make it amenable to the lawful/unlawful distinction. In criminal appeals, therefore one finds the English Court of Appeal creating new ways of rejecting its own past decisions, where those decisions now appear unjust. In doing so its converts injustice into unlawfulness making what was previously a lawful decision, but is now lawful but unjust, reappear as unlawful, giving its present decision the authority of both lawfulness and justice.

For science, the paradox created by the authoritative claim to determine what is true and what is false for society is transformed into the binary distinction, scientifically proved/scientifically unproved, or into attempts, such as Karl Popper's, to distinguish what is 'scientific' from what is 'unscientific' or as yet lacking the conditions for recognition of scientific truth. Through this device science may be able to maintain its authority and its separate identity, creating within its own internal operations a distinction which avoids the paradox of simultaneous truth and falsehood.

The paradox with which this chapter is concerned arose original-ly from attempts to give legitimacy to social work intervention in child abuse by invoking the authority of science (see Chapter 6). If science is able to determine what is true, then social workers' deci-sions based upon scientific principles of what is good or bad for children are as close as one can arrive to the truth and therefore carry more authority than any other kind of decision. Problems arise, however, when science itself is observed to be failing to distin-guish truth from falsehood. Where, for example, apparently scientif-ic methods of identifying child abusers manage to produce many false positive and false negative assessments of risk, it becomes highly problematic for child protection agencies to continue to make decisions as if there existed some privileged knowledge or expertise on what is best for children. Yet social workers cannot simply turn their backs on the social problem of child abuse which their own activities have helped to construct. With or without the legitimacy of science they are obliged to continue in the role of protectors of children against harm.

One solution is to place the responsibility for such failures in regu-lation firmly at the door of politics. Policies which have the result of increasing poverty within families or which deny vital resources to those agencies combatting the effects of deprivation may be blamed not only for increasing the incidence of child abuse, but also for mak-ing the task of child protection agencies an impossible one. Yet is it not now time that the idea, made popular by the more critical writers on child protection (Parton, 1985, 1991, p. 146; Frost and Stein, 1989), that developments in social work child protection practices can be explained entirely by changes in prevailing political ideology, itself to be subjected to some critical examination? This is not to say that there is not and has never been any connection between social work practice and political influences. What needs to be questioned rather is the belief that programmes generated in the political system are able to control events and impose order throughout society. In insisting upon the supreme power of politics these analyses underes-timate the capabilities of other social subsystems, such as law, eco-nomics and science to construct their own environment and to include politics within that environment from their own (and not political) elements. While politics may help to create the environmen-tal conditions in which science, law and social work operate, it does not have the capacity to dictate the internal operations of these sys-tems or the relationships that may develop between these systems.

This chapter then challenges the popular belief that the practices, and the justifications for the practices, that exist within those social organizations concerned with the protection and prevention of harm to children are explicable simply by reference to unbridled political power, creating a universally accepted social reality which obliges every other social system to dance to whatever ideological tune happens to be in fashion, be it welfarism, legalism, socialism or new rightism (Luhmann, 1977, 1989; Teubner, 1992; King, 1993; King and Schütz, 1994; King and Piper, 1995). It may be true that these social systems need to pay attention to the social acceptability of their performance, particularly, these days, in terms of the results claimed for their decisions, but this is very far from maintaining that political ideology is the final arbiter of truth or efficacy.

What this chapter suggests, therefore, is that any analysis of societal evolution requires some recognition of the ways in which social systems themselves generate, through their communications, a self-identity for both internal and external consumption. It starts with Niklas Luhmann's proposition that an important aspect of this process of system-identity construction results from the existence of paradoxes at the foundations of the system and the need for systems to develop strategies to prevent these paradoxes rising to the surface and so undermining their operations (Fletcher, 1985; Luhmann, 1988). This chapter concentrates first on one specific paradox arising from the role of certain institutions in making decisions with the express ambition of promoting the future well-being of children. On occasions these decisions involve removing the children from their families, which is the single social institution associated with the safeguarding of children's interests and the promotion of their welfare.

THE PARADOX OF CHILD WELFARE

Who knows today what is good or bad for children? How is it possible for institutions designed to promote children's welfare to rely on anything other than a self-generated version of what that welfare consists of? In order to observe these problems of system identity we shall travel straight to the front line of child abuse prevention and the problem of determining in advance whether a child is likely to be abused. According to the author of a comprehensive work on the subject:

Because child abuse is a vastly complex human problem, we have not been able to develop a perfect enough understanding of it for successful prediction. At the moment we are unable to predict with accuracy who will and who will not abuse.

(Cohn, 1983, p. 171)[3]

In those situations when social workers are faced with the problem of whether to remove a child from the home, predictions are also extremely precarious. Nobody can know with any degree of certainty what will happen to the child once he or she is removed. Nor can they predict what would have happened had that child remained at home. Statistical studies are of little help, since, although they can provide some indication of the probabilities of certain events, they are unable to calculate with any accuracy whether this or that particular child's removal will be more or less damaging to the child's physical and mental well-being than leaving the child in his or her home. It may be that in a very small number of cases involving extreme violence or neglect, the conclusion that the child will be seriously injured and permanently impaired, unless removed, is inescapable. But in the vast majority of instances, all that social workers and child care experts can do is to make informed guesses using evidence of past situations involving that child and other children as a basis for making predictions for the future. Moreover, it is impossible to know whether the child's future life away from the home is going to be better or worse than a future within his or her natural family. He or she might, for example, be materially better off, but suffer serious psychological problems or even, in the rare case, vice versa. Even children who have suffered serious physical or sexual abuse at the hands of a parent may experience long-term emotional suffering from the loss of that parent.[4] The fact that children initially appear to thrive in every possible way after removal does not rule out the possibility that difficulties may arise later.

Similar uncertainties and ambivalences exist where social workers leave the child at home and try to 'work with the family' or even where they simply choose to do nothing. The only difference here is that, if the decision has negative effects for the child, then these are more likely to be noticed quickly, partly because they are often of a visible kind, such as injuries or symptoms of physical or behavioural abnormality, and partly because everyone has been alerted to look out for these signs.

Where the 'harm' to be protected against or prevented is serious physical injury to, or perhaps also the blatant sexual exploitation of, a child by someone living in that child's home, it is relatively easy to reach general consensus on what is good or bad for the child but matters become much more difficult when public anxiety demands action to be taken in less obvious cases of 'possible harm'. One example might be where the perpetrator of the abuse is the mother's boyfriend, who pays irregular visits to the home. It also becomes more difficult once it is admitted that protective intervention itself carries with it the risk of other kinds of identifiable 'harm' which those making decisions about the child's welfare need to bring into the equation. Furthermore, sensitivity to the impressionability of children and the lasting effects of childhood experiences make it necessary to think beyond the immediate short-term results of the intervention and to set them against the medium- or long-term outcomes for a child of removal from the home. Predictions are always fraught with problems. They must depend not only upon the *identified* harm that the child risks in remaining at home, but also upon everything that may happen to that child in the future including possible *unidentified* harms associated with the trauma of discontinuity of intrafamily relationships and disruption of every aspect of that child's life. And this is to say nothing of possible later events in that child's life which might follow indirectly from the decision to remove, such as fostering failures, periods spent in poorly run institutions (Packman and Randall, 1989, p. 109) or even sexual or physical abuse at the hands of staff or other children (Levy and Kahan, 1991).

The magnitude of the task becomes clearer if we look at attempts by clinicians to account retrospectively for a person's present behaviour or state of mind. Such explanations typically invoke a chain of causality which links specific events in a person's past with present mental illness, personality disorders, difficulties in relationships, forms of unhappiness, etc. Yet, however convincing the identification of harms and the attribution of causes may appear for both patient and clinician, they can never be more than interpretations. It would be quite wrong to treat them as if they represented the only acceptable version of 'reality'. The point is that explaining behaviour is always a matter of interpretation. Interpretations have necessarily to select from everything that is known about people's past and present situations. Yet even to call these interpretations 'objectivity' assumes, first, that everything that could be known about the past is available to the interpreters and, second, that the sum total of all possible interpretations available within society has been placed before advisers and decision makers.

Nor is this the end of the problem of explaining behaviour, for interpretations do not appear out of the air. Rather they depend on the availability of concepts of meaning and understanding. These may range from formal theories to what we call 'common sense' explanations, meaning the spontaneous, unanalytical accounts of events in our lives and the lives of others. Let us take as a relatively simple example the insightful account of a young man who had been sexually abused while in care.

> In 1988, Cleveland hit the news headlines. Child sexual abuse was being discussed everywhere; on the telly, in the papers, at work and in shops. For a time you couldn't get away from the subject – it didn't have much of an effect on me at first, but eventually my life was shattered by the media focus on child sexual abuse. The past which I believed was dead and buried, I then had to face every day. *I had been a victim of child sexual abuse as a child in care, but had never thought of myself like that, because these words and attitudes did not exist in the 1970s.*
>
> (Fever, 1993, p. 4, emphasis added)

The interpretation of his present unhappiness, therefore, is based upon the concepts, which were unavailable at the time when the event (now identified as traumatic) occurred. Furthermore, it would have been quite possible for the young man to choose another interpretative framework to explain his present predicament, such as a religious one, which might perhaps attribute his present suffering to having turned his back on God. What makes the sexual abuse interpretation more valid is not its inherent truth or correctness, but its prevalence in 'the media'. What may have seemed at first sight a relatively simple empirical task of pinpointing those past experiences which have resulted in the present unhappiness, now becomes a matter of huge complexity involving the selection of an interpretative framework from among those which are socially available and acceptable, and the application of this framework to selected events from the young man's memory, which itself, as we know, distorts and selects.[5] If one now considers the position of a person seeking not only to explain the past, but also to prophesy the future in the light of past events, it becomes clear that this will necessarily involve not just all the problems already set out, but the additional difficulties of using current explanatory concepts to predict whether events will or will not occur in the future, and anticipating the likely consequences of these events on the well-being of the child. Yet this is precisely the impossible task that social workers, courts and child care experts would have to confront each time they had to decide whether or not to remove a child from its family, were they seriously to engage in truly 'scientific' decision making. It is true that generalized social values ought to be of some of help in identifying what risks ought to be regarded as potentially harmful to children at any particular time, but in modern society these beliefs are far from consensual. There is no generally agreed rank order of harms to children; nor is such a list ever likely to exist. In the final analysis, therefore, subsequent events and the consequences for the child are probably the only way of knowing whether the decision to intervene was a good or bad one.

The paradox for social work's self-image as the promoter of child welfare, therefore, stems on the one side from the impossibility of performing this task in any reliable 'scientific' manner, given these inherent problems of harm identification and prediction. On the other side lies the inconceivability of admitting that the task is indeed impossible, for to do so would threaten the very existence of this social identity and be likely to cause immeasurable damage to general social morale (to say nothing of the morale of social workers), such are the collective anxieties in our society produced by the prospect of children being damaged and corrupted by those adults charged with their care and welfare.

Of course, other social systems, such as politics, economics and law may well be confronted with the issue of child abuse and neglect. If they accept the construction of the problem by child welfare science within their own meaning system, they are likely also to find themselves infected by the paradox. The results would be similar to those which follow the spread of a computer virus. Within a very short time much of the energy expended in these institutions would become devoted to finding ways of handling the paradox which now exists within their own operations and appears to threaten their very survival. Fortunately, however, these systems are sufficiently complex and sophisticated to avoid importing social work's predicament wholesale. What happens, rather, is that the problem of child abuse is reproduced in terms that are amenable to the system's communications and operations. For politics it becomes a problem of governments demonstrating that they are able to govern, for economics, it is a problem of obtaining returns for the deployment of resources, for science, it is a problem of finding the truth, and for law, it is a problem of determining what constitutes unlawful behaviour.

Yet this does nothing to repair the damage to social work itself and to society's morale caused by the paradox's appearance. Unlike computer viruses, paradoxes cannot simply be eliminated and their future appearance prevented by introducing anti-viral programmes. Nor can they be solved through any logical processes, for, by definition, paradoxes are not amenable to this kind of solution. Straightforward denial of the paradox's existence is, of course, out of the question, as this would run the serious risk of drawing attention to the very dilemma that needs to be hidden. The best that can be hoped for, therefore, is that some way will be found of concealing the paradox. Such paradox-concealing must involve the avoidance of any hint of the paradox's existence in the system's future communications. Probably the most successful method of concealment for any system is to construct for itself a social environment in which the issues that gave rise to the paradox either do not appear or appear in a totally unproblematic way. This will entail major changes in the way the system constructs its own identity within this newly-constructed world.

Some social subsystems are quite capable of achieving this through the kind of proceduralization of the truth criterion that Habermas has identified, where theoretical and empirical issues are replaced by issues of procedure which then provide the criteria for testing truth validity claims (Habermas, 1984, 1985; Raes, 1986; Preuss 1989; Teubner, 1989). This has the effect of immunizing the system against criticism that it is failing to perform the impossible task that society expects of it and which it still claims to be capable of performing, since new realities have changed the nature of the task, while maintaining the appearance that nothing has changed. The hybrid or eclectic nature of social work, however, makes such proceduralization difficult, for its procedures for truth validation derive not from its own elements, but from other meaning systems, such as science, medicine and law. In the United Kingdom over a period of twenty years a profusion of highly publicized 'social work errors' (Howitt, 1992) where predictions and prevention had clearly failed to protect children, effectively ruled out science or medicine helping social work to deal with its paradox problem, so the task was left to law.

Now law's capacities for reconstructing society's contingency problems as issues of lawfulness or unlawfulness, so avoiding the need to learn from experience, are well known (Luhmann, 1985, 1988a, 1989; Teubner, 1989). Its ability to 'deparadoxify' its own operations have also been reported by Niklas Luhmann (1988a). Less well appreciated perhaps is law's tendency in the furtherance of its own lawful/unlawful distinction-operations, to provide other systems with the means of solving their paradox problems, where these problems become an irritation within law's environment. Yet the recent history of child protection in the United Kingdom stands out as clear evidence of the inventiveness of law when faced with a threat, not directly to its own operations, but to the credibility of non-legal communications on which law depends for the effectiveness of its own operations and communications. The irritation to the legal system in such cases is not simply of the kind which can be soothed away by some conflict-resolving decision of the courts. Rather, the very structure of the communicating system on which law depends has to be reconstructed within law in such a way as to restore its authoritative status and thus its usefulness to law. Yet, as we have seen, law may achieve this objective only through its own lawful/unlawful distinctions.

LAW THE GREAT HEALER

Nelken (1990) was surely right when he called law 'the great concealer', but where the future of the concept of children's welfare, on which British child law depends, was in danger of imploding through the revelation of the paradoxical nature of welfare-identification institutions, law has also revealed itself as the great healer, helping society and other social systems to come to terms with the perennial contingency problems surrounding children and their future. After all, was it not law which in the late seventeenth century constructed the notion of children as incompetent beings, in need of the protection first of the monarch and then of the courts against exploitation of their property by unscrupulous guardians (Thane, 1981, pp.14–15)? Did not law later come to the aid of the institution of marriage as the perpetuator of family fortunes by recognizing as a legal concept the notion of paternal authority and so prevent inexperienced heirs from committing the unpardonable sin of marrying for love?[6] By the early years of this century, had law not made a major contribution in reformulating childhood as a period of vulnerability and irresponsibility, requiring protection from violence and exploitation?

In the task of determining what is lawful and unlawful behaviour for and towards children law has always been obliged to make constructive use of whatever systems of attributing value to such behaviours happened to be available at the time. When Christian morality gave way to scientific empiricism as the method of establishing truth in society, law did not lag far behind. It could soon be seen using science in its own decisions about what was good or bad for children (Sutton, 1981). Within this century the legal system has been able to call upon specialist child experts within the new social institution of social work. These experts claimed the capacity to analyse 'the child's needs' and predict the outcomes for the child of different forms of treatment and different emotional environments. To some observers law's task might have been interpreted as doing no more than lend its authority to the experts' solutions for meeting the child's needs and promoting the child's welfare.

For a short period half way through this century it seemed as if this approach would work without a hitch; lawfulness and unlawfulness effectively became at this point virtually indistinguishable from true/false and healthy/unhealthy as identified by the agents of children's welfare, namely social workers and specialist child experts applying their 'scientific' and 'medical' knowledge of what was good and bad for children. However, the illusion that law could solve its decision making problems concerning children's best interests by directly importing external medico-scientific knowledge was shattered by the gradual discovery that many children, whose needs had been assessed and identified according to modern medico-scientific practices, had failed to fulfil the predictions that had been so expertly forecast for their future well- being (Howitt, 1992). The disillusionment which brought the paradox of social work claims of child harm prevention and welfare promotion rushing to the surface also caused a tidal wave of accusations of ineptitude, arbitrariness, 'tyranny' and the infringement of individual and family rights (Taylor et al., 1979; Morris et al., 1980).

Since the validity of legal decisions do not depend upon the consequences of those decisions but only upon law itself (King, 1991; King and Piper, 1995, p. 18), there was no question of the legal system being held responsible for these failures. Nevertheless, law found itself in an awkward position, for there was no denying that it had lent its authority to the social workers and medical experts who claimed to be able to treat children for their delinquency and 'maladjustment'. Having so recently welcomed medico-scientific knowledge on what was best for children into its own programmes, it now found its own operations in danger of being infected by that paradox that was proving so destructive to the claims of social work and child medico-scientific welfare expertise.

So law began setting in motion the well-established deparadoxifying strategy of reconstructing those aspects of social reality which are causing problems in ways that exclude any mention of the paradox. The medico-scientific criteria by which social work wished to evaluate its operations (and which had caused such serious problems of compliance) came, therefore, to be replaced by the legal test of lawful or unlawful. Social work was to be judged not so much by its ability to offer a safe and healthy environment in which children could thrive, but rather by its efficiency in investigating cases of child abuse and producing evidence for the courts to evaluate and by its compliance or non-compliance with rules and regulations, procedures and guidelines that the legal system would so copiously produce. Law, the great healer was able to reduce the problem to manageable proportions, while law, the great concealer, simply hid from sight the insoluble problem of determining children's future welfare in the face of indeterminacy and uncertainty. The paradox problems of social work simply disappeared from view in law's mist of reassuring realities. Children could be protected, individual and family rights respected and truth guaranteed without ever considering the problematic nature of promoting children's welfare through spasmodic and individualized social work intervention.

It was not simply a matter of 'proceduralization' in the Habermasian sense (Habermas, 1985), for law did not merely substitute procedural tests of validity to what were previously normative or moral issues. It was not merely that it offered its protection to social workers who kept to the legal rules. Rather, law additionally constructed for society a well-ordered meaning world of inter-professional cooperation in which, for example, 'welfare' and 'justice' became compatible and obtainable goals,[7] courts of law revealed objective facts, and children's needs and interests could be readily ascertained and presented in court by people with the appropriate professional skills and qualifications.

The situation was not, as some writers seem to be suggesting, one of law simply bullying social work into accepting its tutelage.[8] The 'enslavement' that took place was confined to child welfare knowledge, which law exploited for its own ends. The relationship between the law and social work systems was much too reciprocal and symbiotic to be described as 'enslavement'. Law, as we have seen, evolved from its own elements those interpretative concepts that would enable social work to avoid public disclosure of its paradoxical nature and, at the same time, these concepts were able to enhance law's identity as the ultimate arbiter of what was good or bad for children. This is not to suggest that this was a deliberate rescue operation on law's part. Systems are not capable of such consciously motivated acts. Even lawyers, who are capable of acting in a motivated way, did not set about restructuring social work in the same way that the liquidators of an insolvent company might reorganize that company as 'a going concern'. This rescue operation depended rather on the co-evolution or 'structural coupling',[9] the synchronization of the operations of law and social work around the social problem of child abuse, so that communicative concepts which were generated by one system were available for use by the other. This transfer from one communicative system to the other in turn depended on the existence of media which would give both law and social work the appearance of commonality of purpose. One of the key media was that of rights.

THE LANGUAGE OF RIGHTS

The rhetorical notion of rights with its resonances of freedom from oppression, of resistance to the power of 'the state' had proved itself a powerful political banner for the exploited and disadvantaged ever since the French Revolution. During this century rights claims of particular social groups were a regular precursor for change and reform. Given the claims of social workers that their medico-scientific training made them better able than parents to make judgments on children's well-being, it was only a matter of time before those families who saw themselves as the victims of social work arrogance started to claim that they too had rights. 'Parental rights' and 'family rights' soon became rallying cries for all those who felt that they had suffered injustice at the hands of social work. The response of social work was to claim that it represented 'the best interests of the child', which, according to eminent psychoanalysts (Goldstein et al., 1973) had to take precedence over the rights of parents and families.

It was in the field of juvenile justice, however, with its spectacle of bewildered children, who had committed relatively minor criminal offences, being taken off by social workers to assessment and treatment centres, that the claim that social workers represented children's interests first became rather difficult to sustain. Following the celebrated *Gault* case in the United States Supreme Court,[10] the rights of the child in criminal cases came to be equated with 'due process', that is with guarantees of procedural safeguards for any child accused of a crime, including representation by lawyers at a formal hearing.

In the field of child protection, the claim that social workers promoted children's interests appeared rather stronger, particularly in the light of so many highly publicized cases of parents or step-parents who had killed or seriously injured children in their care.[11] Yet, as we have seen, disillusionment with the assertions of medico-scientific knowledge led to a growing loss of confidence among social workers as to their ability to promote the welfare of individual children through their decisions. For a time it seemed possible that social work could change its image by applying some vague, external notion of children's rights to its own operations. An article appearing in the *British Journal of Social Work* in 1976, for example, seemed to be using the notion of children's rights in an attempt to make social workers aware of and responsive to their own fallibility.

> Rights also include the right not to have help and Social Workers tuned to the ideas of a community approach will appreciate the importance of protecting people from the unintended, but perhaps unavoidable ill- effect of intervention in their life.
>
> (Parsloe, 1976, p. 88, emphasis added)

For social work practice, it was only a short step from this acceptance of the notion that families had rights which on many occasions conflicted with expert opinion on what was best for the child, to the major concession that in certain cases the family's rights should be preferred over expert opinion on what was best for the child. This call for a more reflexive and more self-critical social work combined with social workers' existing self-doubts could only add to the identity confusion. Very soon social workers were to find themselves being forced unwillingly into playing the role of *the enemies of family rights* while lawyers increasingly came to be seen and increasingly saw themselves as rights' protectors (Taylor *et al.*, 1979; Morris *et al.*, 1980; Giller and Szwed, 1983).

This reduction of child protection, sustained by Article 8 of the European Convention on Human Rights – 'the right to respect for . . . family life' – to a contest between rights-holders, namely children, parents and families on the one hand, and *rights-chal-lengers*, the child welfare professionals, on the other, may be seen as a pre-coding essential to law's subsequent reformulation of social work and child welfare. In all innocence, lawyers may have defined their task simply as one of translating political guarantees into pro-cedural safeguards to give parents (and their children) a 'fair hear-ing',[12] but, as we shall see, the effect of their work was to reconstruct child welfare itself as a social field in need of, and amenable to, legal ordering.[13] Children, the rights-holders, would be transformed from citizens and subjects to litigants and clients. Children's suffering would become an opportunity for legal argument and legal action, using the language of rights and rights infringement. Such construc-tions may well be functional for the maintenance of social order and confidence, but they have the disadvantage of excluding alternative, more complex, analyses of the same social events.

THE POLITICAL VERSUS THE AUTOPOIETICAL

Of course, it would be perfectly possible to interpret these changes in child protection policy and practice in a political way. One could see, for example in the appointment of eminent judges and lawyers to the roles of chairing child abuse inquiries, a strategy by a right-wing government to 'individualize' child abuse by identifying indi-vidual error and so distract public attention from their own policies, which were damaging the family structure (Dingwall, 1986; Wroe, 1988; Hallett, 1989; Parton, 1985, 1991, Chapter 3). In more general terms, it seems perfectly valid to interpret the 'emergence of legal-ism' as 'evidence of the collapse of the political consensus upon which the institutional fabric of the welfare state was so dependent' (Parton, 1991, p. 195). Yet these political interpretations have to steer a difficult course between determinism on the one side and conspiracy theory on the other. Not all of them succeed in avoiding these dangers.

There is no doubt, however, that political factors (along with economic factors) played an important part in producing a social environment in which legal and social work institutions performed what they saw as their respective roles. An important part of these roles, as we have already seen, was to respond to changes in the political or economic climate in ways that would permit them to continue to function in accordance with the identity that they had constructed. This is rather different, however, from suggestions that these institutions were driven by political or economic necessities.

A potent criticism that could with some validity be directed against the type of autopoietic analysis[14] that we have so far undertaken is that it tends to 'animate' or 'personalize' law, making it appear an actor in the process of social evolution. 'Anthropomorphism' of this kind which attributes thought and motivation to abstract communicative systems would be inexcusable if it could not be supported by reference to actual social events. Up to now we have tended to deal in a semi-historical way with general trends in the relationship of law and social work. We can bring these abstractions a little closer to the kind of concrete empirically-based findings that many socio-legal scholars today demand by looking at events that have recently taken place in Scotland. In 1989 the kind of dramatic paradox surfacing that had plagued social work in England moved north of the border. Later, after public fury with the social workers and a public inquiry chaired by a senior Scottish judge, Lord Clyde, it emerged to threaten the Scottish system of Children's Hearings. As a case study in legal deparadoxification let us turn to these events in Scotland.

THE ORKNEY SCANDAL AND ITS AFTERMATH

By the time that the Orkney Inquiry Report was published in 1992, the 'rescue' of social work in England and Wales had already been completed with the introduction of the Children Act 1989 which, as Parton points out, consolidated the transformation of social workers into investigators and 'risk managers' within a legal construction of what was harmful to children and how they should be protected against such harm.[15]

In the light of these events in England it was significant that the official remit of the Orkney Inquiry concentrated not on how best to protect children against sexual or ritual abuse, but the operations of the local authority and the decisions of the social workers, courts and Children's Hearings in removing and detaining nine children (Clyde, 1992, para. 1.3). The official response to the crisis, therefore, was to frame it in terms of the decisions of individuals and the policies of the agencies involved in removing and detaining children and this is how issues continued to be constructed in the press, in the Report of the Inquiry (Clyde, 1992) and in the debates following the report's publication.[16]

When, therefore, in early 1993, Lord Clyde spoke at a conference on the aftermath of the Orkney affair, the dramatic events which gave rise to the inquiry,[17] and the variety of concerns and anxieties that they aroused concerning the sexual abuse and corruption of children in a small isolated community, by newcomers to that community, had already been subjected to legal filtering. They had now become transformed into one dominant issue: what procedures and practices in Scotland should determine decisions as to whether or not to remove a child from the home and detain that child away from the family?

To begin with, Lord Clyde was able to reassure his audience that the difficult task of exercising 'discretion' or 'professional judgment' in decisions about what was best for the child (the infamous paradox) could be resolved by 'following guidance' and that this guidance should place emphasis on the need for *clear evidence*. 'Some guidance should be possible upon the occasions on which the discretion should be exercised. Such guidance should include provision emphasizing *the need for clear evidence* to justify the operation . . .' (Clyde, 1993, p. 22, emphasis added).

This same issue of evidence was taken up later at the same conference by Lord Justice Butler-Sloss, author of the Cleveland Inquiry Report which had examined allegations of sexual abuse being made against a large number of parents. She saw the crucial test as one of legal proof, maintaining that: 'There was in Orkney, as in Cleveland, no interdisciplinary approach to the problem, no consideration of widely accepted principles of good practice . . . a lack of consideration as to whether the allegations could be proved . . .' (Butler-Sloss, 1988).

She informed the audience:

> There are three situations of children. There are children who have been abused and you can prove it, and *those children sooner or later you will be taking away from home*, unless you can produce a good system of protection for them in their own home. Then there are children who haven't been abused – you have to be careful that you recognize *they have rights*. Then there are also the children who may have been abused and you can't prove it. . . . But a solid, calm assessment that you can't prove the allegation and *you won't be helping the child in such a case by taking it away from home and sending him back again*.
>
> (Butler-Sloss, 1993, pp. 55–56, emphasis added)

The message to the Scottish social workers present at the conference was clear. It was not simply that acting precipitously without adequate proof of abuse is unlawful, but that it was the strength of the evidence rather than anything else that would provide them with a test of the likely effectiveness of their intervention in promoting the child's well-being. Children's welfare may remain a matter for social workers to promote, but the way the concept of 'welfare' was to be established had undergone a considerable transformation from the days when medico-scientific expertise was called upon to decide where children's interests lay. It had emerged from this transformation as something amenable to legal definition and to management by the legal system.

Cynics might be forgiven for thinking that for government bureaucrats the problem was how to bring the Scottish system of child protection into line with that operating south of the border. But for many of the social workers present this must have been a reassuring message. Some good, it seemed, had at last come out of the disaster of the Orkney crisis. By keeping to guidelines, principles of good practice and, above all, to the legal test of *clear evidence*, they would escape censure and, what is more, could convince themselves that they were acting in the child's best interests. If the social worker's role had at one time been that of helping families solve their problems and promoting children's welfare by offering knowledge and expertise, it was apparent to everyone that it was now primarily concerned with protecting children by assembling evidence for the courts to evaluate (Cooper *et al.*, 1995). A further major stumbling block in the way of the acceptance of this message in Scotland still remained, however. Instead of courts, which could be relied upon to reinforce the performance of the social workers' protective and investigatory tasks, there were Children's Hearings, which still saw themselves as part of a network of agencies involved in solving family problems and deciding where children's welfare lay.

RECONSTRUCTING THE SCOTTISH CHILDREN'S HEARINGS

The Scottish Children's Hearing System, which had won praise throughout the world for the relaxed and informal way in which it dealt with children who had admitted committing crimes, and with their families, was, in its handling of child abuse neglect cases, now under attack for the very features which made it so successful in the management of delinquency cases, namely its flexibility and its free-dom from the formalities and constraints of the legal system (Asquith, 1983). After the Orkney affair the hybrid nature of the hearings had become a matter of controversy and contention. On the one hand they were responsible for decisions which in other jurisdictions would have been made by courts of law, while, on the other, they were not officially courts but rather panels of lay people whose exclusive concern was the welfare of the child. Their role was often presented as that of a mediator between social work agencies and the family in an attempt to find a solution to the child's 'prob-lems'. This 'problem solving' orientation was clearly out of phase with a legal approach which conceptualized parent–child, family–social work and child–social work relations in terms of rights and duties. It was also incompatible with a notion of child protection based on risk management rather than meeting unmet needs. Previously, the hybrid nature of the Children's Hearings had been subjected to some disapproval. Some critics had pointed out that Children's Panel decisions in offence cases were often 'unjust' in that they contravened the principles of proportionality and fairness between offenders, and that the children who came before them risked losing their liberty (by being sent to a children's home under a residential supervision order without any of the procedural safe-guards usually afforded to adult offenders) (Asquith, 1983; Adler, 1985). Yet they had successfully resisted all attempts to impose for-mal legal procedures[18] and legal representation upon them.[19] The delinquency side of the hearings' work might have seemed at first sight a much more likely candidate for reform along legalistic lines than its child abuse and neglect work. However, the total separation that was theoretically possible in criminal cases between the finding of guilt by the Sheriff's Court and the Panel's 'disposition' of the young offender according to the principle of 'the child's welfare' insulated hearings to a large degree from pressures for change.[20] There were major differences between these cases and abuse and neglect problems which made it much more difficult to defend the hybrid nature of the hearings in the case of the latter.

To begin with, parents had not normally participated in the delinquent act. Although they might have been seen as part of the problem, potentially they were also part of the cure, if only they could be recruited to the task of controlling and disciplining their offspring in ways that ensured that the child committed no further offences. Second, the split between fact-finding and disposal was far less easy to achieve in cases of child abuse than in delinquency cases. In determining 'the facts' the Sheriff's Court had to make difficult decisions about the nature of 'harm' and 'children's welfare':

> The role of the court is no longer adequately distinguished as that of determination of facts. In judging the evidence in cases of abuse and neglect, the courts are in some degree involved in defining what are minimum standards of adequate parenting.
> (Lockyer, 1992)

Similarly, the hearings in these cases found it difficult to confine themselves to finding the appropriate disposition without looking at 'the facts' which had given rise to social worker intervention and the finding of 'case proved' in the Sheriff's Court. According to a paper published by the Association of Directors of Social Work in Scotland:

> In cases of child protection a process of review and arbitration between differences is tending to replace open ended discussion and initiation of solutions and services, which the system originally envisaged. . . . Today hearings are more likely to involve adjudications between representations being made to it, rather than a more open minded search for common ground.
> (Association of Directors, 1992, para. 63.3, quoted in Lockyer, 1994, p. 125)

Since finding the 'facts' in these cases almost always involved an examination of parental conduct, some re-examination at a later stage by the Children's Panel in their task of deciding what was best for the child was inevitable. Whenever this occurred, it was extremely difficult to prevent the parents from raising again objections about the nature and seriousness of the abuse and their role as perpetrators, which had already been aired and dismissed before the Sheriff. This in turn paved the way for demands that parents be adequately represented at the Panel Hearings in order that their rights and interests, as well as those of the children, might be protected.

A second set of problems arose out of the procedures for dealing with emergencies, where social workers had removed the child from the home on an *ex parte* 'place of safety' order and now required confirmation that they could retain the child in care.[21] In practice, as long as the hearings dealt predominantly with offence cases, there was little use made of place of safety orders. This was certainly the case during the first decade (1971–1981) following the introduction of the Hearing System, when the number of abuse and neglect cases coming before the hearings was in single figures. Over the second decade, however, this number steadily increased with growing societal concerns over child abuse, until today it represents the majority of cases referred to Children's Hearings.[22] Although no official figures are available, social workers' applications for Place of Safety Orders, it would appear, have risen in line with the increase in abuse and neglect cases coming before Sheriffs and Children's Panels. Moreover, there is good reason for believing that, as social work practice has shifted from needs provision to risk management, the sudden removal of the child becomes increasingly a moral response to 'bad parenting' or a 'shock tactic' to try and bring parents to change their behaviour – for example, in leaving young children alone in the home – rather than what is strictly necessary to save the child from immediate harm.[23] Furthermore, as an increasing proportion of parents now challenge social workers' actions in the court, choosing to contest the allegations in the Sheriff's Court, so the pressure for social workers to prove their case also increases. In anticipation of the courtroom battle ahead the sudden removal of children becomes a legal weapon in hands of social workers and police to obtain evidence, for example from interviews with the child, or to preserve evidence that they have obtained by, for instance, preventing parents from influencing the child to retract allegations (Clyde, 1992).

To those Reporters and Panel Members responsible for the workings of Children's Hearings, it must seem that their belief that gentle persuasion and good will on all sides can find solutions to families' problems is constantly being hidden from sight by the smoke from the gunfire of the legal battles going on around them. There, parents and local authority social workers, each represented by their lawyers, are given every encouragement to fight over the evidence, and protect their rights and what they see as the child's interests. It is hardly surprising that Lord Clyde should find it incongruous that Children's Hearings should be asked to determine upon what he saw as an issue of the legality or illegality of place of safety orders. In the midst of such pervasive legalism the claims of Panel Members that their only concern is the welfare of the child may seem lame and lacking in conviction. What about the wording of the Act? What about the rights of the family? Even if the Children's Hearings have until now restricted lawyers for the parents to an advisory and supportive role, the hostile emotional climate and adversarial mentality that exists after children have been removed forcibly from their parents makes it extremely difficult to hold the line against pressures for parents to be fully represented by lawyers acting on their behalf.[24]

The arrival on the Scottish scene of children's rights lobbyists, ostensibly there to promote children's autonomy and the voice of the child in all decisions concerning his or her future, has not helped matters one little bit. The strategy of these 'children's rights police' is to wave the *United Nations Convention on the Rights of the Child* in the face of any official inquiry or law reform body, referring to it as 'international law' which, since ratification by the United Kingdom in 1991, has to be obeyed (see Chapter 7). They make it their business to ensure that government agencies and courts not only know of the Convention's demands, but that they are also familiar with their interpretation of the way that these Articles apply to the local situation.

The Scottish Child Law Centre in Glasgow has been particularly energetic in this regard. The argument pursued relentlessly by the centre was that the procedures of the Scottish system of Children's Hearings were in flagrant breach of Articles 3, 12 and 37(d) of the Convention and therefore, in order to remedy this situation 'the appointment of a Child Advocate should be mandatory for every child involved in children's hearings'.[25] As a concession to the unique nature of the hearings, the existing Safeguarders – who are at present appointed to befriend older children and represent their views at the Children's Hearings in an informal manner – should be developed into Child Advocates to advise all children who come before the hearings of their legal rights and to represent their interests at the hearings.[26]

Two opposing views now emerge from the debate over what should happen to hearings concerning the legality and continuation of place of safety orders. The one sees the answer in the Sheriff, who, as a qualified judge, is portrayed as better equipped than Children's Panels to unravel the facts and handle the claims and counterclaims of social workers and parents concerning the legality of the child's removal and continued detention. The other argues that, where social services wish to keep the child in care, the matter should be referred to the Children's Panel, the specialist forum for deciding where children's welfare lies. This would permit, as at present, a continuity between the present and future determinations on the relations between the child and the family. Yet in the present climate of legalism, retaining these decisions in the Children's Hearings would inevitably involve concessions to the children's and parent's rights advocates. The legal representation and increased formality that the rights' advocates demand run the risk of changing the nature of these hearings, bringing them much closer to courts of law. Furthermore, it is unlikely that they would stop at the place of safety hearing. Already the Scottish Child Law Centre is calling for advocates to represent the child at all Children's Hearings. Indeed, there seems no logical reason, once the need for legal representation and formal protection of rights has been accepted in principle, why it should not be considered appropriate in the case of every child and every parent coming before the hearings.[27]

In the aftermath of the juridification of social work as a solution to fill the gap between promise and performance, it seems inevitable that the hearings will be unable to sustain a mediation role. Indeed, changes in social work practice had for some time past been making this role increasingly difficult. Individual case workers no longer came to the Panel ready to listen to the parents and discuss with an open mind what steps might be possible to promote the child's welfare. Instead, a social worker appears more as a representative of social services, often after a case conference, which having considered all the evidence, has empowered the social worker to argue for a particular order in respect of the child.[28] Arbitration has tended to take over from mediation (Association of Directors of Social Services in Scotland, 1992). It is a mistake then to see the invasion of legalism into the Children's Hearings, the representation by lawyers and increasing formality, as denoting the beginning of the end for the philosophy on which the hearings were founded. Where abuse and neglect cases are concerned, the end began a long time ago with the juridification of child protection social work. The imposition by law of the notion of *legality* as the criterion for assessing the validity of child welfare decisions, described earlier in this chapter, with its emphasis on rule-obedience, procedural rights, evidence and proof may have rescued social work (and society) from its crisis of confidence by concealing the paradoxical nature of its decisions, but at a high price. The price has been the construction of child abuse and neglect as primarily a legal issue creating legal problems for resolution by legal decision making processes.

CONCLUSION

Although it may be possible to trace the development of this juridification of social work from the first child abuse public inquiry, *Maria Colwell* in 1974, through to the Children Act 1989 and the present upheavals in Scotland, there was nothing inevitable or predetermined about it. Child-protecting social work is not pre-programmed to turn itself into evidence collection and risk management based on the legal criterion of proof. This has not happened in other European countries.[29] Other social institutions involved in children's welfare, to be sure, all have to deal from time to time with paradox problems. Yet they appear to have found ways of paradox concealment which do not involve calling in the law on a regular basis to launder their operations and remove the stains of professional failure by substituting legal criteria for the system's own values. Teachers, for example, are not (yet) obliged regularly to justify their decisions (exam results, entry criteria, etc.) in courts of law. Doctors do not spend their time, before deciding upon a course of treatment for a child, accumulating legally admissible evidence in anticipation that their decisions will be challenged if things go wrong. Yet both these professions have the capacity to inflict irreversible damage on children. To argue that neither of them involves the infringement of parental and children's rights and so avoid the need for systematic legal regulation is simply to go round in circles, for it is only as a result of the juridification of child care that society now perceives the issue in terms of these rights and their infringement. Ultimately, one might seek answers to the questions posed by juridification of child welfare in Anglo-Saxon countries in such culturally-specific factors as a traditional suspicion of the state and state intervention, a strong concept of individual rights and an idealization of 'the child' and 'the family'. Add to these the hybrid, eclectic nature of the knowledge informing social work decisions and practice, social work's historical dependence upon government funding and susceptibility to direct political and economic pressures, and the dependence of social work on the approval and support of other systems for its intervention/non-intervention decisions become apparent. It is able, furthermore, to make little of its successes, but is constantly having its failures exposed to the public gaze. All this adds up to a formidable list of complex factors which together go some way to account retrospectively for why social workers in Britain have found it particularly difficult to develop therapeutic practices for the child and its family. It may also go some way towards explaining why it became necessary for law to rescue social work both north and south of the England–Scotland border.

This is not to argue that the juridification of social problems is always bad for children. Obviously, there are gains and losses. Some criticism is needed, however, where the losses are concealed or swept aside by self-interest or by delusions as to what can be achieved through law's operations. In the Scottish system, for example, the kind of mediation that the Children's Hearings were able to perform may at one time have played an important function in healing wounds and laying down a basis for future relationships between social workers and family. This has now been lost, largely through the construction of child abuse as a predominantly legal issue. Moreover, law the great concealer is well able to hide from sight its own paradoxes. Making its distinctions available to other systems and subjecting the communications of these systems to legal scrutiny may be just two techniques among many for deflecting attention from these paradoxes and guarding against the problematization of law itself. As Niklas Luhmann has pointed out, the legal/illegal distinction replaces for law the much more problematic and historically fraught notions of justice and injustice (Luhmann, 1988b). Observers wishing to embarrass the guardians of the legal system need only ask how it is that law knows what constitutes justice for children and what constitutes injustice.

NOTES

1 N. Luhmann, 1988b.
2 See Luhmann, 1988b, p. 160.
3 Alasdair MacIntyre (1981) provides a useful general discussion on the problems associated with predictability in the social sciences. See Chapter 8, 'The Character of Generalizations in Social Science and their Lack of Predicative Power'.
4 Wallerstein and Kelly (1981), for example, claimed to demonstrate that a child's need for an absent father after the divorce and separation of his or her parents was not related to the quality of the relationship that existed before separation.
5 I am not suggesting here that these operations of selection and application necessarily occur in that order. The selection of 'facts' as salient could just as well pre-date the availability of the child sexual abuse framework or the two events could be simultaneous.
6 Blackstone in his 1765 *Commentaries on the Laws of England* wrote:

The power of a parent by our English laws is . . . sufficient to keep the child in order and obedience. He may lawfully correct his child, being under age, in any reasonable manner; for this is for the benefit of his education. The consent or concurrence of the parent to the marriage of his child under age . . . is now absolutely necessary; for without it the contract is void. And this also is another means, which the law has put into the parent's hands, in order the better to discharge his duty; first, of protecting his children from the snares of artful and designing persons; and next, of settling them properly in life, by preventing the ill consequences of too early and precipitate marriages.

7 Lord Fraser, addressing a Scottish conference on child abuse, stated:

Welfare without justice is ultimately no welfare and indeed justice without welfare is scant justice. The system must be a careful intertwining of justice and welfare at every stage. It must be designed to provide the best justice and the best welfare and to prevent either one jeopardizing the other. We must 'go for gold' in both.

(Asquith, 1993, p. 40)

8 King and Piper, 1990, p. 29. See also Parton, 1991 for a discussion of the relationship between law and social work.
9 See pages 186 note 27
10 *Re Gault* US (1967), 527.
11 For example, Maria Colwell and Jasmine Beckford.
12 These included the right to challenge in court any social work decisions concerning visits to their children, the according of party status to parents along with the right to legal representation at hearings for legal aid.
13 See also Chapter 7 for a detailed discussion of children's rights as international law.
14 Teubner (1992), King (1993) and King and Schütz (1994) provide an account of autopoietic theory particularly as it relates to legal operations.
15 See Parton, 1991.
16 See further discussion later in this chapter.
17 The affair began in November 1990 with the removal from their home under Place of Safety Orders on the island of Orkney of seven children belonging to one family, following the allegation by one of the children of sexual abuse. In February 1991, after more allegations had been made, this time concerning what appeared to be an organized ring of sexual abusers involving the children and parents of other families and the local church minister, nine further children were removed. These nine children were then questioned by police and social workers. The issue of their detention under a Place of Safety Order was brought before an informal Children's Hearing, which in Scotland decides on issues of children's welfare, once the facts of the case had been established, and was not empowered to consider the

legality of the removal or the merits of the case against the parents. The Panel therefore referred the matter to the Sheriff's Court and on 4 April the Sheriff, having listened to claims by the lawyers that the proceedings were 'incompetent' because of technical irregularities in the removal and questioning of the children, released all nine children to their parents, and so ended the affair without any examination of the validity of the sexual abuse allegations.

The outrage of the parents and their supporters at what they claimed was the totally unjustified removal and detention of their children by social workers, now given legitimacy by the Sheriff's decision, was taken up by the press. Calls for a public inquiry were heeded by the Secretary of State for Scotland and the inquiry was set up under the chairmanship of a senior judge, Lord Clyde.

18 One exception may be found in the Rehabilitation of Offenders Act. This treats any admission of guilt made by a minor at the hearing as a recorded offence for the purposes of the Act. Its requirement of a formal admission by the minor contrasts with the informal nature of the rest of the Panel Hearing.

19 The British Government, for example, had entered a reservation to its ratification of the UN Convention on the Rights of the Child, which excluded the hearings from those Articles of the Convention requiring the legal representation before courts of children deprived of their liberty. The instrument of ratification stated:

> Children's Hearings have proved over the years to be a very effective way of dealing with the problems of children in a less formal, non-adversarial manner. Accordingly, the United Kingdom, in respect of Article 37(d), reserve its right to continue the present operation of children's hearings.

20 Adler (1985, p. 77), writing from a children's rights perspective, points out:

> According to the rhetoric of the Scottish system of juvenile justice, the anticipated consequences of the different available disposals are the overriding criterion in all decisions made on behalf of children. The reality is very different, for very often that actual decision is the only one available in the circumstances, or it may (despite the contrasting rhetoric) be taken on grounds involving societal needs of legal requirements.

21 Under the existing arrangements, set out in Sections 37–40 of Social Work (Scotland) Act 1968, a Place of Safety Order to remove a child from his/her parents may be made by a Sheriff (or in exceptional cases, a Justice of the Peace). If the child is then retained, the law requires the Reporter to bring the matter before a Children's Hearing for consideration within seven days. This *first lawful day hearing* may release the child to the family or grant a further warrant ordering that

the child should remain in a place of safety until (in contested cases) the Sheriff's Court has decided whether the facts for compulsory intervention exist and (in uncontested cases or cases where the Sheriff's Court has found the case proved) a hearing has considered what long-term steps should be taken to promote the child's welfare. Although there is some confusion over the longest period that a child may be detained without a full hearing before a court or Children's Panel, the maximum is probably 91 days and then only if the case has been back to the Panel on two occasions and to the Sheriff's Court on a further two occasions. Where a Children's Hearing issues a warrant for further separation of the child from the family, the parents may appeal to the Sheriff's Court and the appeal must be heard by that court within three days.

22 While only very few children are separated from their families for longer than seven days under a warrant issued by a Children's Hearing, the number of Place of Safety Orders applied for and granted by Sheriffs and JPs is remarkably high compared to the situation in England and Wales. One reason for this is the difference in the legal criteria. In England and Wales, since the Children Act 1989, children may only be removed and detained under an emergency protection order where the child is likely to suffer imminent and significant harm. In Scotland by contrast the existence of one of the abuse or neglect grounds for referral is sufficient for the granting of a place of safety order. These include the belief that a criminal offence of child abuse or neglect has been committed against the child or another child in the same household or that the child is likely to be caused 'unnecessary suffering or serious impairment of health because there is, or believed to be . . . lack of parental care'.

23 This was certainly true of the use of place of safety orders in England, according to a study carried out for the DHSS Review of Child Care Law.

24 The Scottish Child Law Centre (1993, p. 91), for example, while opposed to place of safety hearings being transferred to the Sheriff's Court, argued that legal aid should be available for parents to be represented at Children's Hearings.

25 This proposal follows closely the ideas of Professor Donald Duquette of the University of Michigan Law School (see Duquette, 1987). The Child Advocate, while not necessarily a qualified lawyer, should 'be accountable to an independent board, child welfare commission or children's rights commissioner (Marshall, 1992, p. 22) and perform all of the roles normally associated with a legal representative. Furthermore, where any disagreement arose between the Child Advocate and a child of at least 12 years old, the child should have the right to choose 'a personal legal representative'.

26 It is worth mentioning that according to a recent unpublished survey carried out by Elaine Sutherland of Glasgow University School of Law, almost half the Safeguarders who at present attend some Children's Hearings as 'befriender' of the child and spokesperson for the child's interests, are solicitors.

27 The Scottish Office in its recent White Paper (1993) proposes a mix-
   ture of these options, retaining the Children's Hearings as the forum
   where arguments for the continuation of an emergency protection
   order will normally be examined, but giving to parents the right of
   appeal to a Sheriff as soon as an order has been granted (The Scottish
   Office Social Work Services Group, 1993).

28 Andrew Lockyer, an experienced Panel Chairman, writes:

> Social workers have become to a large degree 'bureau professionals',
> who are increasingly the purveyors of collective departmental policy
> and case judgments. Individual social workers at hearings are thus
> more inclined to be viewed as inflexible and constrained partici-
> pants – not open to influence by families, or amenable to discuss
> alternative disposals proposed at hearings.
>
> (Lockyer, 1992)

29 In France the number of cases going before the children's judge is
   much higher than in British courts, but the jurisdiction exercised by
   the judge is based for the most part upon medico-scientific criteria. In
   Sweden child care cases tend to be dealt with by administrative rather
   than court decisions, while in Holland the juvenile courts pay much
   more attention to the issue of the child's welfare than to matters of
   proof and procedure (see King and Piper 1990, Chapter 8).

Chapter 4

Doing good for children – mission impossible?

INTRODUCTION

The specialization and diversification of functions in modern society has made it virtually impossible for social helping institutions to
formulate their activities around particular moral principles. These
institutions may operate as if they took the mission of doing good
extremely seriously. On the other hand they experience enormous
difficulty in putting this mission into effect in their operations. This
difficulty arises in part from what we have already identified as the
absence of any universal or absolute notions of morality in modern
society. Furthermore, assessments of 'good' or 'helpful' (or for that
matter, 'evil' and 'detrimental') cannot simply be assumed from the
organization's operations, since these operations produce only decisions on whether or not to intervene, and, in the case of intervention, what form the intervention should take. Only observing
systems, such as law and science, are in a position to judge the value
of these decisions and usually retrospectively in terms of their
results. Criteria for success based on these judgments inevitably
become reconstituted within the programmes of the social helping
system, which treats them as offering a guarantee of success for
their helping operations. The helping system is then left with the
task of continually defending its decisions in face of competing
claims for moral authority or for truth and validity invoked by
other ideologically based or functionally differentiated systems.

The difficulties encountered by assertions of being able to identify and promote children's welfare or 'the best interests of the child'
are no different from the general claims of being capable of helping
or of identifying and promoting 'welfare'. Doing good for children
presupposes the possibility of doing bad for children, and in the

absence of some universally accepted distinction of good/bad for children which does not ultimately depend upon medical, scientific, economic or legal criteria, or upon ideological claims of benefit/deficit, notions of what is good and what is bad for children have to be constructed in a self-referential way within a system which society expects to be capable of making such distinctions.

While God may do no wrong, but is recognized as working in mysterious ways, the benefits of which may not be immediately apparent, the same is unfortunately not true of social workers. They cannot claim immunity from external observation. Even if social work might wish to maintain an identity founded on the distinction of good/bad for children (or families or even society), the most it can achieve under the present conditions is the distinction, intervention/no intervention in the lives of people. Furthermore, whether intervention occurs and, if it does, the form that it takes, are likely to be determined and legitimated, as we have seen in previous chapters, not by moral considerations, but by criteria constructed within legal, political, economic and medico-scientific systems. It is these systems that decide what constitutes lawfulness, value, social justice and health for children.

Because the ambition of doing good has meaning only where evil is readily and constantly identifiable, the effect is to create closure around the helping intervention or practices of helping organizations and the professional activities of social workers. Once taken out of its religious context 'doing good' loses its capacity to recognize evil through self-reference. Evil becomes what others identify as evil, which is then reproduced within the system of social work as the target at which 'doing good' should be directed. In relation to children, one needs only to substitute the term 'harm' for that of 'evil' and 'promoting the welfare of the child or the child's best interests' for 'doing good' and the problems of child protective social work become apparent.

THE EMERGENCE OF THE CARING PROFESSIONS

What have been called 'the caring professions' began to emerge in Northern Europe and North America during the nineteenth century, relatively late in the process of industrialization and urbanization. A lack of confidence in the ability of impoverished families to care for their own was nothing new, as the Elizabethan Poor Laws in England had borne witness. But the idea that there should be laws and secular institutions charged with promoting care for the casualties of society had to wait until the essential conceptual prerequisites were in place. These included the revolutionary idea, born out of the Enlightenment, that all people living within identifiable geographical boundaries could constitute something called 'a society' (or 'a nation'). From that point on it was a relatively short step to the belief that 'society' could be regulated. The later enfranchisement of almost all the adult population helped to bring into existence not only the possibility of regularly changing governments, but also the concept that the government or 'the nation state' was capable of making rational, informed decisions that would bring about improvements in society and that failure to make decisions, or making decisions which appeared to have negative consequences, could result in the downfall of governments.

Before society came to be seen as the nation state and governments as the guardians of the economic and moral health of that state, it had of course been possible for British philanthropists such as Dr Barnardo, Octavia Hill and William and Catherine Booth to regard themselves as members of a community which had obligations towards its weaker and more vulnerable members. But there was a clear distinction between individual charitable action inspired by religious or secular moral principles and the much later intervention by governments which took upon themselves the responsibility for alleviating poverty and assisting the victims of adverse social conditions. To quote David Garland:

> In the terms of the state's official pronouncements and representations . . . there was an important distinction drawn between the spheres of public and private life, a distinction that, with a few special exceptions, the economic, moral or religious welfare of individuals was strictly a matter for private arrangement.
>
> (Garland, 1985, p. 45)

Individual philanthropists and charitable organizations were to devote themselves to the rescue and care of fallen women or the child victims of cruelty, neglect and exploitation, like those whom Dickens had described in *Oliver Twist* and *Little Dorrit*.[1] Yet, any notion at this time that the abuse of children was in some way a problem *for society*, the solution to which was in part intervention by national governments, is from the retrospective view point of the twentieth-century observer conspicuously absent.[2]

As long as caring for the destitute and exploited children of the poor remained in the hands of the church and those charitable organizations which depended upon the generosity of a handful of private benefactors, there was no need for their operations to find justification in anything other than religious principles and moral ideals. To quote Philp (1979) 'in charity work the workers represented the humanity of the privileged to the poor and the essential "goodness" and social nature of the poor to the privileged' (p. 84).

It was only in the latter half of the last century (at least in Britain and America), when charities started to see themselves as independent collective enterprises, that they were to draw upon rational, economic justifications for their work – the powerful Charity Organization Society, for example, was described by its promoters as 'a charity applying business principles' – and upon the new forms of knowledge discovered by the social sciences. It was these expanding areas of new scientific knowledge which made it possible for what were once considered moral deficiencies and defects of character, such as viciousness and drunkenness, to be removed from the realm of individual responsibility or individual misfortune and constructed either by psychology and psychiatry, as, for example, the legacy of adverse childhood experiences, or by sociology as 'social' problems; that is, as the products of a society that was itself defective. This process was accelerated when in the early part of this century private child-rescuing and other charities began to work alongside the state organizations of police, courts and prison service.

Historical accounts of the foundation of the welfare state have often assumed that prevailing social conditions and the inspiration of a handful of tireless social reformers and insightful politicians was all that was needed for raw capitalism to transform itself into a caring capitalism. For observers of communicative systems, however, such accounts do not overcome the problem of explaining how society was able to change itself in such fundamental ways. For these systems theorists, as we have seen (Chapter 1), modern society's identity, its conception of itself, is the product of the operations of its normatively closed, differentiated systems, which provide the authority and justifications for social communications. Yet, paradoxically, it was the normatively autonomous, self-referring nature of theses separate systems, each of them capable of coding the external world in accordance with its self-generated selections, which gave modern society its coherence and its unity. Far from providing a cohesive image of society, however, each of these systems of politics, law, economics and science, as we have discussed in previous chapters, inevitably developed its own *internally generated* version of reality and its own *internal* processes for reproducing this vision of society and guaranteeing its future (Luhmann 1977, 1982, 1986a). For law, society and its future were to be secured through the development of universally applicable lawful/unlawful judgments on people's behaviour. For economics, society's salvation lay in the productive regulation and distribution of money and property. Science was engaged in the business of rejecting the untruths of the past and discovering new truths for the future improvement of human existence. Within politics, there was a growing expectation that political power would be dedicated to the solution of each country's, and later the world's, social problems.

THE REGULATION OF SOCIAL NOISE

The optimistic notion that present society was quite capable through its rational operations of repairing any damage caused by its own past and of acquiring the means to avoid future damage, found resonances, therefore, in all of these systems. The difficulty in putting these solutions into practice, however, was that each system's vision of what constituted society was restricted by its own selectivity, that is by its specific binary coding of its environment (Luhmann, 1986b, 1987, 1989 and 1990). Metaphorically, each was able to see itself and other systems only in the blinkered terms of its legal, political, scientific or economic selections. Both together and separately their communicative codes produced within each system versions of modern society which reduced anything that did not have meaning for them to the status (or rather non-status) of 'noise'. Thus, noise consisted of whatever could not be explained using the programmes available to the system, but nevertheless had to be acknowledged as existing. It was, for example, conduct which was neither lawful nor unlawful, but was considered within politics as requiring regulation and control. For medical science it was the bizarre behaviour of those people were clearly ill, because they were incapable of rational thought or regulating their own lives, but whose bodies produced no symptoms of any illness that could be treated in a scientific manner. 'Noise' consisted also of people, such as beggars, gypsies and tramps, who were not part of the labour force and had no fixed position either socially or geographically and, therefore, no existence in present society or stake in the development of society's future. At times it would also include people whose stated beliefs or lack of beliefs placed them outside what the politics of government and opposition regarded as the parameters of political activity. It could also be found in irrational and uncontrolled outbursts of emotion which, since the time of the Enlightenment, had appeared so often to confound predictions, corrupt reasoned decision making and thwart even the best laid projects. Included in these were what we now refer to as 'domestic violence' and 'child abuse', which tended to be seen as products of drunkenness and a failure of men to control their instincts.[3] These, however, tended to be regarded as beyond the scope of government and, while they might have represented 'noise' for the family, it was only in the early years of this century that they came to be seen as matters of *social* concern, that is, concern that the 'noise' should be reduced to social order, that it should be understood as having meaning.

In former times, noise, the unknowable, could simply have been left for religion to decipher. It could remain unknowable and attributed to God's will or to the devil's works or to some other cause or being existing outside society. It soon became apparent, however, that for modern society this possibility was no longer present or present in only a very limited way. Michel Foucault's works on madness and sexuality offer historical accounts of the way that various aspects of the unknown became knowable and, in a certain sense, governable (Foucault, 1977, 1978, 1979). Yet it had to await the arrival of postmodernism before the very indecipherability of 'noise' was finally recognized as possessing the quality of meaning.

Seen from the perspective of autopoietic systems theory, the mere recognition of the existence of noise by any one of society's function systems anticipated a commitment to reduce noise, if not by that system itself, then by one or more of the others. Within law, for example, science was constructed in a way that made comprehensible to law much of what law, applying its limited code, of lawful/unlawful, found meaningless.[4] Moreover, the demands that each system made of the others and their interdependency on the meanings produced by these others, resulted in internal programmes being developed within each system specifically for the purpose of presenting its internal operations in forms that could be reproduced by other systems on their terms and thus these meanings could become 'communicated', externalized and generalized. In science, for instance, these were scientific 'theories'; in law they took the form of judgments, verdicts and court reports; in politics, they were legislation; while in economics they took the form of the many and varied ways of indicating economic performance. This process, together with the increasing speed and efficiency of the communications media, produced expectations of continual and potentially limitless expansion in what could become known and understood.

Seen in the light of these general but at the same time highly specific hopes and aspirations, the arrival of the professional social worker on the scene begins to take on retrospectively an air of inevitability. The increased opportunity for the reduction of noise and the transformation of unspecified dangers into knowable and eventually controllable risks (Luhmann, 1993) that social work's exploration of society's noisy underworld appeared to offer could only intensify society's optimistic expectations of its own future. The function of social work or social help (Baecker, 1994) would be the inclusion within society of those people who had hitherto remained outside its perimeters.[5] 'Social problems' could thereby be reconstituted as 'people's problems' and these problems could in time be resolved through helping and therapeutic intervention. Buoyed up by the enthusiasm that greeted each new development in its activities, social work was able to float freely for a time in the spaces provided for social problem-solving. This was a time when optimism abounded and the spaces were soon filled by a wealth of new ideas for the creation of a risk-free society where social problems were to be soluble through the co-operation of all social institutions guided by 'discoveries' in the social and behavioural sciences, and those individuals who created problems were to be returned to the straight and narrow through treatment and therapy. Paradoxically, however, the very act of intervention became increasingly likely to stigmatize 'victims' in such a way as to jeopardize the very social inclusion which the system was supposed to achieve.

THE PRINCIPLES OF SOCIAL WORK

Given this early enthusiasm and the rapid growth of professional social work over the first sixty years of this century, it was not surprising that people began to talk of the 'principles of social work', as if social work had achieved a form of coherence and distinctiveness which separated it from society's existing function systems and allowed it to see itself as an observer of those systems and, what is more, a highly critical observer. While at first these principles of social work may have reproduced within new settings the religious or charitable virtues of kindness, generosity, and altruism, they soon took a very different direction, drawing upon the knowledge derived from the new social and psychological sciences to create the possibility of a different society where each of these organizations would operate for the benefit of all humanity. In a similar manner, personal suffering was also seen as remediable through the application of treatments and therapy derived from newly acquired insights about the human psyche and a faith in the ability of people to restore others to mental health and stability through a professionalized altruism.[6] Professor Paul Halmos was able to claim that the principal function of the newly created 'personal services' was 'to bring about changes in the psycho-social personality of the client'.[7]

The rapid growth of professional specialist helpers and counsellors over the first sixty years of this century helped social social work achieve a form of coherence and distinctiveness which made it independent from those systems which society regarded as authoritative and allowed it to see itself as an observer of those systems. Its programmes were able not only to guide and inform its intervention decisions, but also to reconstruct other systems as playing a powerful role in creating social problems and, therefore, as being morally obliged to assist helping intervention to resolve the problems that they themselves had helped to create.

People who were engaged in helping others in the eighteenth and much of the nineteenth century were likely, as we have seen, to explain their behaviour either in terms of the Christian virtues of kindness, generosity, and altruism or in the language of moral imperatives – the inherent rightness of doing good, of setting an example to others and assisting those less fortunate than oneself. From the second half of the nineteenth century, however, they were increasingly likely to justify their work by drawing upon knowledge and techniques derived from the social and behavioural sciences (including economics). Even if, as Halmos's book, *The Faith of the Counsellors*,[8] suggests, this evocation of rationality and science might have concealed compelling personal motives, this individual motivation was recognized socially through the existence of scientific evidence which indicated that doing good was *scientifically good* in that it improved in scientifically accountable ways both people and society. These evocations of scientific knowledge to justify (and rationalize) the work of the emerging helping professions echoed the 'scientific' approach of the great social reformers, such as

Sidney and Beatrice Webb and their fellow Fabians, who saw professional social work as an essential part of the apparatus of reform that would contribute towards the construction of a society very different from the one that existed. With the help of science and an army of professional carers, what once had been dismissed as noise would reappear as harmony.

While social scientists were able to construct an image of themselves as independent, objective observers of society, even if it was admitted that their observing operations might at times change what they were observing, social workers could not, of course, confine their role to that of observer. On the contrary, the communicative system of social work was founded on the premise of 'social action'. It had a right (and, later, even a legal duty) to intervene in any situation where its knowledge and techniques, according to its own evaluations, were likely to improve matters. Social work was to operate in a self-reproductive manner, therefore, according to a binary code of intervention/non-intervention, where intervention could result only in improvement for those towards whom it was directed, for society as a whole and for social work itself.

If these ambitions turned out to be unachievable, it was not simply the result of insufficient political will or economic resources, poor communications or management, although each of these explanations hold obvious attractions for political analysts of both the left and the right. Explanations which draw attention to social work's parasitic nature go some way to making explicit the problems. Hodges and Hussein (1979) refer, for example, to the need of social work to graft 'itself onto education, medico-hygienic practices and to the penal and the judicial'. This, however, might lead one to believe that social work in some way 'lived off' other systems and that its success or failure depended upon the continuing health of these host systems. In practice its relationship to these other systems had, as we have seen, been a symbiotic one, with social work making comprehensible and controllable the 'noise' that the host system's operations had simultaneously created and rejected as lacking in meaning. There was no possibility of these systems 'failing' without the whole of society 'failing'. What was equally unthinkable at that time was the failure of social work to make noise comprehensible to one or more of these systems.

THE MANAGEMENT OF SOCIAL WORK

In the second half of this century in Britain, a long series of child abuse scandals occurred (starting with Maria Colwell and ending with Cleveland and the Orkneys), as a result of which social workers were portrayed in public inquiries and in the mass media as inadequate and unreliable decision makers. These events provided social work with ample opportunity to observe itself and construct an identity which constantly emphasized reflexivity, self-awareness and self-improvement. We must remind ourselves, however, that we are talking here of social systems and not of conscious systems and that social systems, unlike people, are limited by their selectivity, their inability to see beyond the limits set by their distinctive coding of their environment. For social systems any attempts at 'self-improvement' must necessarily be applied by their internal operations to their own processes and procedures. This does not deny the influence of external influences, but rejects a simple input–output model which sees systems responding in a direct way to external events. It rejects even more firmly the idea that social work was in some way 'taken over' by politics, law or managerialism (Clarke *et al.*, 1994). For social work to remain social work and not become something else it was not only necessary to reassure the public that social workers were indeed capable of efficient decision making, but this reassurance had to result from social work's own operations and not be seen as a subjugation of social work to political, legal or economic demands. If social work was to retain its identity, its distinctiveness from other social systems, it was required, like Baron Munchausen, to raise itself into the air by pulling on its own bootstraps.

The official inquiries that followed these child abuse scandals in Britain made social work pay much attention *to its own practices*, its 'good practice' and its 'bad practice', almost to the point of obsession. Even the briefest examination of the communications which are today generated by and directed towards social work operations, will find an abundance of directives, codes, regulations, checklists and guidance which cover almost every aspect of practice. Official government documents published by the Department of Health following the Children Act 1989,[9] for example, instructed workers on how to go about meeting their responsibilities under the new legislation. These instructions include detailed guidance as to the procedures to be put in place in fulfilling those statutory duties. In investigating and making an initial assessment, for instance, social workers must, according to these instructions, ensure that families are kept informed, they must interview specified categories of people in specified venues and their findings and conclusions must be recorded (Department of Health, 1995, Chapter 8).

In a similar vein, the Social Service Inspectorate[10] was set up to inspect and measure services against 'clearly stated and coherent standards' derived from 'legislation, regulations and guidance and current professional understanding (based on research and professional experience) of what constitutes "good social work practice" and management of services; and what constitutes "good quality services"' (Department of Health Social Services Inspectorate, 1993, p. 1). It stipulates that each local authority Social Service Department is expected to have a clearly written comprehensive child protection policy. It must be based on legislation, regulations, guidance and knowledge of what constitutes a 'quality child protection service' (ibid., p. 33). This policy, it is stated, must be operationalized through written procedures, (ibid., p. 34) identifying which levels of management are responsible for making crucial decisions. Similarly, the Social Services Department, together with the Area Child Protection Committee, is expected to produce a handbook of procedures and to monitor the implementation of those procedures. (ibid., p. 36–37). Social Services Departments must also have clear structures for the management and accountability of staff and quality control systems for child protection work (ibid., p. 38–39). Staff should be taught how to measure the outcome of their work.

Inspections by the Social Services Inspectorate have been designed to measure services against 'clearly stated and coherent standards derived from legislation, regulations and guidance, and current professional understanding (based on research and professional experience) of what constitutes good social work practice and management of services; and what constitutes good quality services' (Department of Health, 1993, p. 1).

The constant emphasis in these documents on the effective management and monitoring of social work practices, far from indicating the kind of grafted relationship with other systems that Hodges and Hussein identified, would appear to present social work as a self-regulating, autonomous professional body capable of an independent, self-sufficient state of existence. Accountability and self-regulation appear as the heroes of this account of the transformation of social work, while management or (as some would have it) managerialism, is the magic potion which has enabled social work to perform this miraculous change of identity, while keeping the principles and objectives of social work with children and their families firmly intact. According to one account of the managerial revolution, therefore, although 'social work was repeatedly penetrated by the administrative processes', this penetration 'seemed necessary if the system were to function properly' (Howe, 1992, p. 505).

Critical observers of these developments, armed with clear ideological positions, have tended to take strong objection to what they see as the imposition of managerial solutions, the transformation of social work into a 'managerialized enterprise' (Langan and Clarke, 1994). Such blatant managerialism, they argue, following hard upon the colonization of social work by law and the new right's attempted demolition of the welfare state, constitutes the most recent in a long series of attacks on social work practice and social work principles. Law, political dogma, the media and managerial and economically inspired reforms are seen as constantly interfering with these principles and obstructing the practical application of child welfare knowledge (Parton, 1991; Pollitt and Harrison, 1992; Langan and Clarke, 1994; Pahl, 1994).

The problem for these critical observers is that the recent management revolution does not attack its target in any direct way. It does not attempt to confront or criticize the therapeutic ideals, altruistic values and social scientific premises on which social work practice is supposedly based. On the contrary, the language of managerialism takes for granted the legitimacy of social work decision making by repeatedly referring to such matters as 'the evaluation of risk', 'determining the quality of services', 'assessment of the child's needs', 'the measurement of desired outcomes', and taking care not to usurp its function by offering any guidance as to the meaning of 'children's welfare' or 'the best interest of the child' or as to how the professionals should arrive at the evaluations, assessments and measurements necessary for efficient and effective decision making.

The bureaucratic language of the Department of Health Social Services Inspectorate and the Audit Commission simply assumes the existence of some sound principles and body of knowledge according to which reliable child welfare decisions may be reached. It is taken for granted that the knowledge for making these judgments is readily available and that all that is lacking are clear, detailed procedures to ensure that the knowledge is put into practice in the most efficient, cost-effective manner.[11] The fact that the many procedural directives offering criteria of success, based on such measurable factors as time and money, may bear little relation to what others, whether Marxian or Christian analysts, psychoanalysts or representatives of other forms of analysis, see as the 'real' or 'true' indicators of children's welfare[12] is not in itself a problem for social work. While it may be a problem for the conscience of individual social workers, even they are likely to appreciate the benefits of certainty and determinacy in their decision making endeavours. In any event, identifications of 'harm requiring intervention' and analyses of 'the kind of intervention' required, the hallmarks of the social work process, are able to continue untroubled by the management revolution in social work. They have simply been transformed by the language of management into such items as 'risk factors' and 'danger signs' to be recognized by social work. Within the communicative system of social work both the managers and the managed, both the critics and the criticized are engaged, therefore, in the exercise of constructing a belief in and an acceptance of social work practice, the intervention/non-intervention decision, as the crucial factor for the protection of children against danger and the improvement in children's lives.

THE SOCIAL WORK ENTERPRISE

Let us pause to consider the nature of the enterprise that social work had set itself, or, as some would argue, that politics had set for social work (Parton, 1991). What amounted to a major change in professional orientation in the first half of this century was, as we have seen, achieved by the simple device of taking psychological and sociological knowledge about families and constructing them in ways which made it appear that these sciences were indeed scientific in a positivistic sense, that is, capable of identifying 'the causes' of social events and of changing their course through informed intervention. Social workers were able to claim that through the application of professional knowledge and skills derived from the social sciences they were able to improve the lives of children, that is, to know what is best for children and to predict accurately what is likely to happen to them. How much more efficient, therefore, for governments to use social workers, not simply as helping hands to repair the damage caused to children, whether by poverty or adverse parenting, but as the identifiers, predictors and preventers of those harms. To quote Nigel Parton, writing as recently as 1991, '[W]ho is to decide what is harmful, how harmful consequences can be avoided and who is to guarantee the absence of harm? . . . it is primarily social work that has this role' (Parton, 1991, p. 214).

Yet we know that the reduction of 'noise' (or in Luhmann's terms, 'danger') through knowledge leads inevitably to an increase in risk, for

> the more we know, the better we know what we do not know and the more elaborate our risk awareness becomes. The more rationally we calculate and the more complex the calculations become, the more aspects come into view involving uncertainty about the future and thus risk
>
> (Luhmann, 1993, p. 28)

Yet, as I have indicated, it was not the historical accident of its association with the behavioural sciences that gave social work its distinctive identity, on which the social workers relied for their professional status, which increased knowledge, but social work practice as helping, therapeutic intervention. In applying knowledge from the behavioural sciences social workers invariably reproduced that knowledge as 'applicable knowledge', that is to say, knowledge that had some practical application in the decisions that social workers were obliged to make in order to protect children.

Such was the pressure upon social work to rescue children from risky situations that in Britain it appeared for a time as if monistic explanations for all forms of child abuse – those based on the abusing family – had resulted, like blood-letting for the medical profession in the eighteenth century (Johnson, 1972, p. 72), in a single therapy, namely the removal of children from dangerous families. It was as if greater awareness of risk had resulted in social work excluding from its practical or applicable knowledge everything that was known about children and their development which did not in some way throw light upon the intervention issue as to whether the child should remain in or be removed from the family. This, it could be argued, was hardly a scientific way of proceeding and it was to lead directly to the child abuse scandals, the subsequent public inquiries and eventually to a disillusionment with science as the principle guide to helping intervention.

One result of the disillusionment with science was that for practical decision making purposes 'risk for children' became simplified to 'risk of criticism of social work' (or of individual social workers). Any uncertainties concerning the child's future could be subsumed within a risk analysis which concentrated upon the harms caused or likely to be caused by intervention going wrong and the need to prevent those harms or potential harms in a way that minimized risk to the decision maker. In this way also the self-referring nature of knowledge concerning harms and risks to children on which social work practice relied, could be effectively concealed.[13] Law was now able to come to the aid of social work by offering a framework for decisions capable of substituting lawfulness and unlawfulness for both scientific truth or untruth or morality's virtue or vice. Through law, failures of parenting, the presence of 'dangerous people' in the home, evidence of non-accidental injury and 'disclosure' of sexual abuse could all be interpreted as indicating an unlawful situation which justified a social work decision to remove the child from the home. In the same way management principles were able to be reconstituted within social work to make risks 'manageable'. According to one commentator, therefore:

> The way the problem was being defined pointed towards certain kinds of solution. The analysis of past failings suggested that success in child abuse work would come by: (i) knowing what information to collect about parents in order to determine whether or not they may be a danger to their children, (ii) systematically collecting that information by thoroughly investigating cases, (iii) processing and analysing that information to decide whether or not children were safe in the care of their parents, and (iv) closely monitoring and re-assessing cases in which children were thought to be at risk.
>
> (Howe, 1992, p. 499)

What was changed was the object of social work's attention which switched from society and its risk-creating systems *to itself* and its own capacity to identify risk situations, predict dangerousness and take steps to intervene and so prevent the potential harm to children. It would appear that the Munchausen therapy of observing itself and admitting its own failures has succeeded in creating a new, autonomous, reflexive, self-aware social work in the place of the over-ambitious, scientifically suspect and politically impure system that existed before the public humiliation of social workers in child abuse inquiries and in the media (see Chapter 3).

The proceduralization of social work

For the observer of systems in modern society what is interesting here is not so much the arguments over the supposed impact, positive or negative, of managerialism on social work, for management can do nothing else but manage and it will be seen as managing either well or badly, but always on its own (measurable) managerial terms. What is interesting rather is the way in which social work has been able to accommodate within its own communications the heavy burden of expectations as society's social problem-solver that law, politics and economics so generously loaded onto it. In the terms of autopoietic theory, therefore, the crucial question for observers of social systems is not what harm management has or has not done to social work principles, but whether social work can be identified as a system producing authoritative communications separate and distinct from the environment in which it operates, and able to make decisions from its own self-generated elements, by reference to *its own past decisions*.

If one searches for those distinctive normative principles in the programmes and practice which provide social work with its autonomy and its separate identity, they are not, unfortunately, to be found where many individual social workers would want to locate them – that is, within the humanitarian values of caring and compassion for one's fellow human beings. Nor do they exist where many academic researchers and supporters of therapeutic intervention would hope to find them – that is, within scientific accounts of what is good and bad, healthy and unhealthy for children, the mentally sick, old people and 'the community'. Rather they are located within and only within social work's ever-changing criteria (or 'programmes') which guide its intervention/non-intervention decisions. The coding of the environment, the process of decision production, itself determines normative principles for social work decisions. In other words, the identity of social work as a distinct communicative system, exists and can exist only in the procedures and processes that it produces for its own decisions. Although individual social workers might well want to take refuge from such a terrifying theoretical conclusion in psychotherapy, politics, religion, money-making, the social sciences, or the legal world of rights and obligations, such moves do not change the essence of social work's identity which is concerned solely with the notion of 'helping' intervention. Observers of such intervention may portray it as right or wrong for

any number of different reasons, but social work can judge its intervention decisions only in terms of its compliance or non-compliance with its own programmes, processes and procedures for
judging what is a proper situation for intervention and what form
the intervention should take.

This is not to suggest that legal, political, economic or scientific
or managerial communications do not influence social work decisions. Clearly they do. The point is, however, that they do not do so
in any consistent or coherent way. Nor is it possible to predict if or
how their influence will continue in the future. In social work decision making, at any one time and environmental setting, one set of
(external) influences may prevail, and, at another time and another
place, a very different set of influences may hold sway. Decisions
about the present and future welfare of children, for example, may
be based on a wide variety of simultaneously existing values. They
may include identity politics – highlighting the child's ethnic, cultural or racial background, and gender politics – empowering women
against male violence. They may equally be based on the ideal of
keeping families together or the important ideal of removing children from corrupting or dangerous people. They may be based on
medical criteria – failure to thrive in physical or mental development. They may be based on legal principles as to whether certain
grounds for intervention have been met and whether legally reliable
evidence exists. Social work itself has no criteria which would
enable it to choose in any systematic way one set of influences as
valid while rejecting the others. Nor does it possess any means of
ranking the different criteria or sets of criteria.

Again, if one takes the example of social work with children and
their families in Britain today, this is not only differently organized
from the way it was organized fifty or so years ago, it is different
both in terms of the way that the issues are presented and in the criteria used to justify and legitimate decisions. Similar evidence comes
from comparisons between the work and attitudes of social workers
in different countries. A recent book comparing social work practices and ideologies in relation to children in France and England,
demonstrates how different cultural environments create not only
totally different breeds of social workers, but totally different
processes and criteria for assessing the value of social work decisions (Cooper *et al.*, 1995).

My conclusion, therefore, will take a somewhat different form
from that of the critics of today's managerialism. It is that there has

never been and there never could be pure and uncontaminated social work principles determining what is and is not harmful or evaluating in some objective scientific or some moral or political manner the value of its work. All that has existed within the system of social work is social work's own self-reproducing programmes for intervention/non-intervention decisions. Talk of managerial interference with social work principles (Langan and Clarke, 1994; Pahl, 1994) or the destruction of these principles by financial attrition or unsympathetic political dogma are in fact complaints that the external truths and value statements which previously served as the dominant or strongest 'interferences' for social work, influencing in an unsystematic and unpredictable manner the way in which social work programmes were translated into intervention/non-intervention criteria, have now changed. Instead of socialism, scientism or welfarism, anti-racism or feminism, we now have managerialism.

Up to a point managerialism is able to help social work avoid the need for such impossible selections and rankings by constructing procedural correctness/incorrectness as the all-important distinction for social work decision making. In other words, the decision is a correct one for social work if the appropriate procedures, such as obtaining a statement of the child's wishes, calling a meeting of all interested parties and informing the parents of the meeting, have been carried out, and incorrect if they have not.[14] Of course, the social problem of abused children does not disappear as a result of these decisions; nor do the individual children concerned necessarily benefit from them, but at least 'noise' has been reduced to the point at which it can be recognized, classified and acted upon and the 'noise-reducing' operations can be seen to work in a rational manner.

THE LIMITS OF MANAGEMENT

Why then should this imposition of management principles as 'good social work practice' cause problems for social workers? Clearly to those civil servants who drew up the many rules, regulations, guidance and codes of practice, there are no problems. Nor are there problems for social work managers whose task of determining 'the right decision' for the child is made much easier by this proceduralizing. For those individual social workers whose motives for becoming social workers had to do with wishing to devote their lives to the welfare of others or a desire to improve society through the sensitive application of social science knowledge, managerialism may present very serious difficulties. Management may be good at structuring organizations in ways that increase their productivity and efficiency, but it is insensitive to any need to make sense of 'noise', where that noise consists of the casualties, outcasts or rejects from other organizations. Indeed, management principles may well operate in ways that reduce the possibilities of treating such social problems as amenable to intervention, simply because including them would decrease the efficiency of the organization's internal operations. In other words the interference of management in social work programmes may seriously restrict the opportunities for other organizations to off-load their 'noise' onto social work, with the result that therapeutic help is offered to fewer and fewer categories of 'victims' and to a diminishing number within those categories. This may eventually cast serious doubt over the capacity of social work to fulfil its task of social inclusion.

One can well understand how it might appear to individual social workers that the space that once existed for 'helping' and 'doing good' has disappeared. Indeed, the saintly virtues of altruism and self-sacrifice and the nineteenth-century ideals of caring and concern for the weak and vulnerable may no longer have any place in the official programmes and practices of social work. To an extent the same is true of the language and concepts of psychoanalysis and the behavioural sciences, which at one time defined the value of the social work enterprise.

This is not to suggest that social workers as individuals are any less likely to be virtuous or scientific than their predecessors, but that the particular form that social work communications (as opposed to personal communications between social workers) now takes constructs an environment within social work where it is unlikely that these attributes will be interpreted in a positive way, unless they are first reconstituted in managerial terms of efficient decision making and effective deployment of resources. Disillusioned social workers may comfort themselves with the knowledge that there are still people who are able to cling on to what were once called virtues and more recently went under the name of 'a social conscience', but these people are unlikely to be social workers. If by some miracle they are social workers, then they should not expect social work to recognize their 'goodness'. It might even disown them.

A similar problem exists when attempts are made to revive the enterprise of basing social work on social science. While within law, economics, politics or the media, scientific knowledge is replaced by 'expertise' – that is, by specialist knowledge which is made to answer the specific questions raised by problems encountered in the application of system selectivity – within social work systems selectivity is confined to the issue of intervention and to the management of social work practice. The truths of the social sciences now enter social work transformed, for instance, into those 'risk factors' which social workers are required to list as signifying danger for children and as guides to effective child protection.

It is not surprising that reports have emerged pointing to the demoralizing effects of the management revolution within social work. Yet it would be an illusion to suggest that a golden age of social work existed in earlier decades this century when helping intervention *really helped*, when therapeutic practices *really made people's lives better*. The struggle that some defenders of the 'old-style', of compassion and belief in achieving a better world through scientific progress, is not, as they would have us believe, a battle for the soul of social work. Social work has never had a soul. All it has had is a capacity to decide whether or not to intervene. The moral, political and scientific values that once informed these decisions, and which have diminished now in their influence, were never undisputed forces for good. Indeed, there were those who maintained that these values were immoral, politically wrong and unscientific. What we are witnessing now in the vociferous protests against managerialism, and in the nostalgia for an idealized past, is hardly the war of independence that the protesters seem to believe they are waging, for to be independent to do good is an impossible goal for social work. The inspiration lies rather in a political ideology which maintains that the past was better than the present and that the future can be better than the present by returning to the beliefs and principles of the past.

Yet in observing these critics of social work's managerial fate we have no reason to be complacent. In its social role, social work is still engaged in the reduction of the 'noise' created by other systems and 'social problems' identified by those systems. Changes in the self-image of social work have followed, and in some sense been driven by, changes in what constitutes 'noise' and 'social problems' for law, economics, medical science and politics and so for society. Altruism, love and kindness may still operate as positive moral attributes in religious and general social communications about children and families, but attempts to translate them into terms which have meaning for society via its social systems succeed only in transforming them into something very different. The resonances they produce within the systems of modern society reproduce them in economic terms as unpaid labour or 'budgetary savings', in law as rights and duties, in science as measurable factors to be subjected to scientific truth-testing, and in politics as attributes that have no place in politics. The only error that the critics of managerialism in social work make is to claim that an earlier version of modern society succeeded in applying moral virtues unspoiled in its social decisions.

NOTES

1 And in the works of many other Victorian novelists and poets. See Brown, 1993, Chapter 3: 'The Exploited Child'.

2 The debate concerning the reform of the Poor Laws between 1795 and 1834 and in particular the prevalent notion that the wholesale relief of poverty would encourage idleness and weaken the workforce and England's competitiveness indicated how far mainstream political thought was at that time from any concept of state welfare intervention. See Poynter, 1969.

3 For example, the introduction of a domestic jurisdiction to the magistrates courts of England and Wales as a response to husbands' violence towards their wives did not take place until the Matrimonial Causes Act of 1878, and cruelty to children did not become a specific crime until the Prevention of Cruelty to and Protection of Children Act, 1889.

4 See Chapter 7 for a discussion of law's reconstruction of psychological and psychiatric communications. Also see King and Piper, 1995.

5 See Dirk Baecker's (1994) discussion of social help as a social function system.

6 The description on the cover of the seminal book by the sociologist Paul Halmos, *The Faith of the Counsellors* published in 1965, encapsulated this spirit of optimism by declaring:

> The twentieth century has seen the emergence of a new secular professional. He is the social caseworker, the psychotherapist, the psychiatrist, the probation officer, the marriage guidance counsellor – *the person whose job it is to help others through personal care for them* (emphasis added).

7 Halmos (1966, p. 5) quoted in Johnson (1972, p. 13).

8 See note 6, above.

9 Such as *Working Together* (Home Office, 1991) and *The Challenge of Partnership in Child Protection* (Department of Health, 1995).

10 Formerly the Social Work Service and prior to that the Home Office Children's Department Inspectorate.

11 Inspections by the Social Services Inspectorate are designed to measure services against 'clearly stated and coherent standards . . . derived from legislation, regulations and guidance, and current professional understanding (based on research and professional experience) of what constitutes good social work practice and management of services; and what constitutes good quality services' (Department of Health, Social Services Inspectorate, p. 1).
12 See, for example, Valentine, 1994 and Kroll, 1995.
13 See Chapter 1 and King, 1995.
14 Howe (1992) writes:

> Once the powers-that-be have written the rules and established the routines, all that the wary social worker and her supervisor have to do if blame is to be avoided is 'go by the book'. Responsibility for failures cannot be attached to the worker if she behaved correctly and ensured that all that should be done was done.

Chapter 5

The James Bulger trial

Good or bad for guilty or innocent children?

INTRODUCTION: CHILDREN AND MORALITY

Reading the newspaper reports of a recent child abuse scandal or of the murder of a child, it is very easy to arrive at the conclusion that we are living in a society where the moral code is a powerful steering programme for society. Even if people may differ in their politics, their religious beliefs, their life-styles, at least all are united in their condemnation of these threats to children. A common surge of emotion at events which cause us fear and anxiety is not, however, the same thing as a common morality. Even a shared belief that steps should be taken to protect all children against serious harm does not answer the important moral questions: 'What constitutes harm?', 'What form should this protection take?' and 'What should happen to people who harm children?' Is the society's morality, for example, the same as that of 'prison culture' which treats child sex abusers as if they were the scum of the earth and subjects them to harassment, beatings, even murder?

One solution is to separate the abuse from the abuser, so that one condemns the abusive act as evil, but seeks humane and progressive ways of dealing with those people who have harmed children. But there is little evidence to suggest that a moral consensus exists for making such a distinction. Indeed, the media reports and analyses following the James Bulger murder, set out in this chapter, suggest that there is considerable disagreement about the correct way to see and treat children who abuse and kill other children. Many of the recent controversies over failures in child protection result from a lack of consensus over the issue of state intervention in the privacy of the family. So, while there may be disgust and outrage at the spectacle of serious harms committed against children, these emotions do not translate directly into some moral code which can be used as the basis for the regulation of the behaviour which is seen as causing these harms.

Placed within the theoretical framework which I set out in Chapter 1, a belief that behaviour towards children can somehow be regulated through the combined operations of different social systems depends upon the construction of a society which has the means to know what these harms are and has the ability to take steps to eliminate or reduce them. These beliefs, and the assumptions about the society on which they are based, become severely tested when confronted with moral dilemmas, such as the killing of a parent by a child who was the victim of that parent's sexual or physical abuse. Any moral judgment of such an event would have to determine the issue of the greater harm which, in the absence of any universal authoritative moral code, has to resort to other means of determining what is the correct judgment. In a society differentiated according to the various functions which allow it to exist and ensure its future, this inevitably involves the application of the distinctions offered by law, science, politics, economics, etc. – distinctions which allow us to conceptualize events as existing within a social world.

In this situation it is perhaps not surprising that the newspapers and the media tend to vent their moral judgments upon those agencies and institutions which they portray as having the responsibility for moral welfare, such as social work, the courts and schools and, of course, families, as if they somehow represented society itself and their failures and inadequacies were symptomatic of the state of society. Such moral judgments tend take these organizations to task as if they were responsible for having allowed the situation which gave rise to the moral dilemma to have arisen in the first place. In the absence of any clear vision as to how to arrive at 'a good society' (except perhaps that of returning to an idealized past), it is these institutions and organizations which become the evil to be reformed and transformed into more virtuous versions of themselves, so that 'the good society' comes to be seen as depending upon guarantees of their future virtue. While this does nothing to resolve the original moral dilemma, it does allow it to remain unresolved and so hold out the possibility of some future resolution. In the meantime, social organizations may occupy themselves with achieving greater efficiency in the production of legal, economic, medical, political and scientific decisions.

The argument offered in this chapter, then, is that while personal morality may or may not act as a guiding force in the lives of individuals there is no longer any possibility of regulatory decisions being taken at the social level on the basis solely of some overriding ethical principle, even if attempts may be made subsequently to justify them on moral grounds. The chapter concerns the killing of a very young child by older children. It traces the evolution of social communications which begin by creating the image of a society which is able to respond uniformly and concertedly to 'the evil' in its midst. This image then becomes fragmented as it is necessary for the irritation of 'evil' to be reconstructed in different guises by different social systems to the point where evil becomes 'normalized' and 'institutionalized' as a harm which, given the necessary force of law, resources, cooperation and goodwill may be subjected to effective regulation.

THE JAMES BULGER MURDER TRIAL

In February 1993 the severed, battered body of 2-year-old James Bulger was found beside a railway line in Bootle, Merseyside in the north-west of England. It later transpired that two 10-year-old boys, Robert Thompson and Jon Venables had abducted James from a shopping precinct and led him to the railway where they stoned him, beat him with a metal bar and left him unconscious lying across the track. The two boys were subsequently found guilty of murder in an adult court and sentenced to indefinite detention. The following analysis of social communications following the murder seeks to account for the outbreak of moral outrage and collective guilt that swept through the newspapers and broadcasting media.

The problem with moral panics

In modern society, where communications usually need to conform with notions of rationality in order to be treated seriously, it is difficult to understand how the age-old struggle between good and evil could still become a prevalent image for making sense of particularly disturbing events. In the hands of critical theorists this could be seen as the result of deliberate government invocation of 'evil' to create public anxiety which the government then proceeds to calm with the introduction of ever-more repressive policies and with reassurances that their new policies or the reinforcement of old policies are now able to control the evil. If one abandons, however, the notion of 'moral panics',[1] the way may be left clear for an approach which does not rely upon the dubious attribution of ulterior political motives to every outbreak of collective *angst*. Following this alternative path, the common tendency to create morality plays out of social disturbances may be interpreted as no more or less than a blind preoccupation with society's future health. Accordingly, the moral condemnation which rapidly followed the trial of the two 10-year-old killers of James Bulger, with its 'demonization' of children, may now take on a rather less sinister appearance. The image now is of a community grappling with its anxieties first by using archaic language in an attempt to alert itself to the enormity of the threat and, only subsequently, by reducing and generalizing it as *a social problem*, which, given time, fits neatly into the pre-existing categories – products of society's systems – for rational problem-identification and problem-solution. According to this system's theory perspective, the difficult and interesting task for social observers, however, should not lie in describing how something called 'society' manages to give itself a fright and then reassure itself that all is under control. It is rather in accounting for the ways that different simultaneous definitions of and solutions to the same 'problem' – a characteristic unique to modern society – are brought together to provide agreement as to what it is possible to disagree about, and as to the choices available for resolving this disagreement. Moral communications, even where religiously inspired, may play their part in this process, but only to provide us with the fleeting glimpse of an utopia, an unattainable moral universe, the antithesis of the image of society's present state. It will probably not be long, however, before statements of 'the way things are' and 'what needs to be done to make things better' evolve to deal with the problem by restating it in terms which are both comprehensible and reassuringly familiar.

Before we proceed any further, however, a word of explanation for what might appear as detachment and even indifference. In a world in which people exist in a constant state of trepidation about their future it is not at all surprising that refutations of treasured notions about what children are and how they behave should become matters of high risk, calling for urgent risk-avoidance and risk-containment decisions (Luhmann, 1993). To present the consequences of such an event as the death of a very young child at the hands of two other children in the detached terms of sociological theory is not to trivialize the horror felt by the majority of people at this destruction of a child's life. Nor is it to condone lynch-mob reactions or the symbolic transformation of children into monsters. The following analysis seeks neither to inflame these strongly felt emotions nor to hold them up to criticism or ridicule.

The coding of social events

The construction of a disturbing event as a crime does not preclude other meanings simultaneously being attributed to the same event. For an insurance company, for instance, it could be represented in economic terms as indicating need for a payment to a policy holder who was the victim of the crime, a debit to be set against the company's profits; for the health system, it could represent the need for urgent medical treatment for the victim or psychiatric therapy for the perpetrators; for religion it could be a sin, requiring confession and atonement; for politics it may be reconstructed as an occasion to require more powers to demonstrate the capacity of the government to control the situation, or the superiority of its regulatory policies over those of its political opponents.

Although moral communications may attribute a negative value which devalues or degrades those people who appear to be responsible for events which disturb the apparent equilibrium, the assignment of a totally negative value to people is a risky business in a society where any overriding moral authority is conspicuously absent. Until there is some modern way of 'understanding' such people's conduct, moral judgments have to be suspended, at least publicly. At the social level this 'understanding' can come only through the operations of function systems. To condemn a woman who kills her husband as evil on no other basis than that a human life has been ended in a violent manner does nothing to avoid the risk of subsequent coding of the event as 'accidental', 'legally justified through provocation' or the 'uncontrollable act of a mentally sick person'. These second order distinctions are made within each subsystem by attributing meanings derived exclusively from the application of that subsystem's coding of its environment to people or things that are capable of being understood.[2]

It is this absence of some overriding moral authority[3] that makes such cumbersome, two-stage processes so necessary in modern society.[4] Far from offering certainty and security, moral evaluations which pre-empt 'understanding' not only run the risk of subsequently having to be revised, but they are also likely to undermine, by exposing the arbitrary nature of their selections, the epistemic authority of those communicative systems which society has developed to attribute meaning to events. An evaluation of 'good' or 'evil' to the perpetrator before the social significance of the event or the motivation of the actor has been decided by law, risks pre-empting any declaration that the event was not one to which moral assignations are legally justifiable. The moral judgment that a particularly brutal murder was the act of an evil monster tends, for example, to undermine the authority of any subsequent decision that 'the monster' was, according to medical opinion, suffering from schizophrenia and could not in the circumstances be held responsible for his conduct. Such pre-emptive moral strikes may also risk exposing the self-referring nature of the moral code itself.[5] The observer may be surprised to find no supportive authority for its communications other than that which is self-generated or that which relies upon some idealized past or some utopian future.

By contrast, the contribution of the general language of morality, once meanings derived from subsystems are in place, may well have the beneficial effect of reinforcing social consensus and so avoid contests and conflicts of authority between function systems or between one or more function systems on the one side and morality on the other. The authority of law, for example, tends to be weakened if it declares unlawful the theft of papers which exposed corruption among politicians, since politics might well see the theft as a justifiable political (or moral) act. Only if there is agreement between the operations of law and politics on the value that they attribute to the act is it possible to make general moral attributions which avoid conflict between systems, such as 'technically illegal', but 'morally justified'. Law, health, politics, science and religion may all operate as closed, self-referential systems,[6] but they are all dependent upon one another for the production of consistent versions of the causality of disturbing social events and of their authority and ability to contain and control such events. In these situations of dependency moral judgments produced after mutually acceptable 'understandings' may operate as a cement, binding together these varying versions of reality.

In the case of a highly disturbing event, therefore, such as the murder of a young child by other children, which makes its first appearance as an outrage against the moral order, there could well be a sound argument in favour of suspending public enthusiasm for moral judgments. The anger of the crowd outside the courthouse where Robert Thompson and Jon Venables, the two boys, were being tried for the murder of James Bulger, may have found expression in throwing stones at the police van taking the boys away from the courtroom, but the formal denunciation of the killing, its open discussion in terms of the boys' motives and moral responsibility, was obliged to wait until law had determined that this was the kind of conduct and the boys were the kind of people on which it was permissible to pass moral evaluations. Only after society 'knew' that the conduct of the two boys was a crime and not something else, and the perpetrators, according to the law, were criminals, and not something else, was it permissible to indulge publicly in the luxury of debates concerning the existence of evil and, where it was thought to exist, the causes for its existence.[7] Even then, these debates did not flow freely, implicating every possible causal factor, but as I shall show, were constrained in ways that made the causes of the evil appear amenable to the demands of rationality and the existing conceptual apparatus for containment and control. As we shall see, the socially efficient construction of 'moral turmoil' in modern society requires skilful management so that the future appears not so much a 'leap into the unknown' as a choice between two different, known solutions, and a choice that entertains the possibility that one of these solutions may be proved right and the other wrong, or that some compromise may be found between them which will eventually provide society with the best of both worlds. With this in mind, let us turn to the events following the jury's decision that Robert Thompson and Jon Venables were guilty of murder.

Applying the code of the moral

Mr Justice Morland, the judge at the end of the trial of James Bulger's killers, described Robert Thompson and Jon Venables as 'wicked and cunning boys' who had committed 'acts of unparalleled evil and barbarity . . .'.[8] What followed in the mass media was the kind of outbreak of moral condemnation that is usually reserved for the enemy in times of war. 'The Devil himself could not have made a better job of raising two fiends' was how the *Sun* the next day greeted the news of the boys' conviction.[9] Yet, it was not only the popular tabloid papers that indulged in the 'demonization' of the two boys. The same day *The Times* leader was headed, 'The Three Evils'[10] and seized the opportunity to offer a homily to the nation not only on the evil nature of the killing itself, but on the insufficiencies of contemporary ways of understanding children, which failed to recognize 'a darker side [of childhood] which past societies perhaps understood better than our own' and according to which children were 'presumed to be innately good'.[11] The same theme was taken up by Dr Hapgood, the Archbishop of York, who wrote of 'the importance of [the] crime lies in what it says about the potential for evil in children of an age at which innocence was once taken for granted'.[12] For *The Times* leader the legal verdict in the James Bulger case had changed the very way in which the nation perceived children and childhood. Its historical analysis invited its readers to recall a time in the past which understood childhood better than our own modern society. Contemporary society or time present, had, according to the Archbishop, deluded itself into believing in the illusion of childhood innocence, while for him, future time, time after the legal verdict in the Bulger trial, was a look forward to an age when the 'the darker side of childhood' would be recognized once more as it had been in time past. Now that the boy killers had been condemned for what the law proved them to be – criminals and evil – watchful parents would in future be on their guard to protect children from their potentially evil instincts. Janet Daley on BBC's *The Moral Maze* echoed this analysis, when she said:

> We used to believe in the innate evil of childhood and we used to accept that it was the moral responsibility of all adults to keep it in check . . . by dismantling the concept of evil we've effectively disarmed ourselves . . . left ourselves helpless in the ability to cope with it.

For the Archbishop of York recent past time could be described even more precisely as time immediately before the Bulger murder – a time of 'evil imagination', a 'pollution of the mind', 'a mental indulgence with the fascination of evil' – and present and future time, made possible by the Bulger trial, as a time when evil, in the form of the murder, having been exposed and society having expressed its sorrow for what had occurred and made its repentance for its past errors possible, could look forward to better, more wholesome, times. 'If the whole sad story can lead to a greater awareness of the extent to which the so-called "adult" world has entertained evil, played with it, lusted over it, and indulged it,' the Archbishop wrote, 'then James Bulger may not have died in vain.'[13]

This sentiment was echoed in the *Sunday Times* three days later when it reported that 'Parents everywhere are asking themselves and their friends if the Mark of the Beast might not also be imprinted on their offspring'.[14]

The distinction between time before and time after Bulger, which draws upon the image of a society as an ongoing entity with a clearly identifiable past, present and future, onto which time distinctions moral attributions may be superimposed, follows fast upon the legal construction of events. Legal time becomes social time and the problems of temporal distinctions within a moral code are resolved by differentiating between a bad past and a good or better future. The James Bulger killing was coded as a crime as soon as the police made it known that two 10-year-old boys had been charged with James' murder. Once this selection had been made, subsequent events could be divided up according to legal concepts of time, relevance and significance. The reporting of these events in the mass media became structurally linked[15] to legal decisions, as did the Archbishop's religious representation of the world before and after the James Bulger murder. It was these legal decisions and their consequences that laid down the agenda for what could be reported and commented upon as 'news': the decision of the prosecution to play in court tapes of the police interrogation, to call the boys' teacher as a witness, to have the boys examined by psychiatrists and ultimately the decision of guilt and the sentence of the judge.[16] Only when the law had taken its course could a distinction be made between time before and time after the James Bulger case. And this was not the only way in which the legal system's 'understanding' of the killing and its perpetrators was able to facilitate (but not cause) the subsequent moral debate.

In a similar manner, the devaluing of children may also be seen as an attempt to remove or conceal the absence of universal authority inherent in modern society's version of morality,[17] a bolstering of the moral coding, 'bad, but innocent' through its assimilation to the distinction, criminal/innocent, that had already been established by the legal system in its framing of the issue of the responsibility of children for criminal acts. The presumption that children's *doli incapax*[18] could be rebutted by evidence of the child's knowledge and understanding of the difference between right and wrong and the failure of the defence in the Bulger trial to rebut this presumption was a precondition for the subsequent moral dramatization of the murder as the triumph of evil over innocence.[19] As the anthropologist Clifford Geertz tells us, 'the defining feature of the legal process [is t]he skeletonization of fact so as to narrow moral issues to the point where determinate rules can be employed to decide them' (Geertz, 1983, Chapter 7).

Not applying the law

Of course, it is possible to envisage the application of the code of the moral, the evaluation of children as good or evil, as the anxious response to a socially disturbing event, even without the intervention of the legal system depriving Jon Venables and Robert Thompson of the right to be regarded by law as children and even without the ritual of a fully blown (adult) criminal trial. Such a sequence would, however, have risked leaving society in a situation of considerable confusion and uncertainty. If events had followed the alternative course of action, favoured by many countries, of deferring criminal liability until adolescence,[20] this would have been to deny society the opportunity of placing the killing and the two boys within a conceptual framework provided by the legal system. There would have been no trial and no finding of guilt. Any moral judgment would have been speculatively based on an incomplete 'understanding' of the nature of the act and the culpability of the perpetrators. It would have run the risk that at any time in the future information could have emerged, for example concerning the mental state of the boys, that would have cast serious doubt on the wisdom of the moral judgment. In the contest between morality and psychiatry, the relative nature of the moral code would have been exposed; good and bad would have been seen as a product of a moral system, the authority for which was not, as its supporters claimed, society as a whole, but its own self-generated elements.

Likewise, if the two boys had been dealt with according to psychiatric (and not other) coding, for example, as mentally ill or disturbed children with damaged personalities, there could have been a glaring inconsistency between their construction as 'sick' or 'disturbed' and their presentation in the media as the personification of corrupted innocence. Indeed, if mental health rather than law had been applied to the James Bulger killing, it is likely that society would have been presented with an expert diagnosis of the problems that had caused the illness or personality disorder from which the boys suffered and recommended a regime of therapy to assist them achieve mental health and control of their behaviour. In a world where, to put it in the crudest terms, 'mad' usually excludes 'bad', and 'bad' usually excludes 'mad', such attempts to understand the causes of the behaviour of the two boys,[21] based on 'psychological' analyses, would hardly provide the kind of definitive judgments that are required for moral evaluations. How was science then harnessed so that the impression of a moral consensus could be constructed?

The scientific alternative

In psychodynamic accounts it is the conscious and unconscious minds of individuals which become the centre of attention. Time, according to the programmes of psychiatric science, unlike decision-punctuated legal time, is a continuous stream which mediates the lives of individuals and families in such a way as the past controls the present and the present governs the future – the French *en amont* (upstream) and *en aval* (downstream). Where such accounts are constructed with a view to therapeutic practices, time begins and ends with treatment which is usually indeterminate, depending upon the patient's progress. There is no precise moment and no clear decision, such as a finding of guilt or a prison sentence, at which a different kind of time can be said to start for the individual. Mental illness is there developing internally within a person over time. His or her bizarre or dangerous acts are significant only as expressions of this inner turmoil which existed before and continues to exist after these acts, until it is relieved through treatment. Thus, in a world where belief that a person can be possessed by the devil is shared by very few people, a diagnosis of mental illness or a personality disorder does not in itself allow moral messages to be drawn (unless, as was the case in post-Stalinist Russia, psychiatric treatment is a pseudonym for social exclusion and punishment).

Moreover, both psychological assessments and therapeutic practices are normally private rather than public events. There is confidentiality about the identity of clients and patients. While internal communications may be rich in detail and drama, those intended for the outside world tend to be in the form of scientific reports or case studies where personal dramas are reduced to clinical and statistical data and to examples designed to illustrate the causes or responses to treatment of general psychological malfunctioning. One could go so far as to suggest that psychology in general provides an impoverished environment for moralizers.[22] Yet the optimistic message that both clinical psychology and psychiatry communicate is that of increasing powers of prediction and increasingly successful treatment of those suffering from 'internal disorders' which give rise to violent or irrational behaviour.[23] It is the scientific rationality of these communications that makes them immune, or at least highly resistant, to moral judgments.

Science 'enslaved' by law

If the legal system were to be effective in producing for society an unambiguous account of the killing of James Bulger, an account based on apparently rational decisions, which could be converted with ease into simple moral messages, it was necessary for law to construct within its own programmes some awareness of the existence of psychological, or medico-scientific explanations for the two boys' behaviour, but which at the same time did not threaten to undermine the version presented in legal communications. Medicine and science had to be reproduced, therefore, in such a way as to serve legal objectives. In the case of serious crimes the English law, and that of most other European and North American jurisdictions, allows this to be achieved by using psychiatrists or psychologists as the expert determiners of such issues as whether perpetrators were at the time of the crime suffering from a mental illness or were for some reason out of control through (according to the wording of the English law) a 'disease of the mind',[24] or 'abnormality of mind'.[25] In England and Wales, where a case concerns a child of between the ages of 10 and 14, these 'psy' experts may also be used to determine criminal responsibility by answering the question as to whether that child was capable of understanding that their behaviour was seriously wrong. It was in both these roles, and not as purveyors of an alternative account of events to that produced by law, that the experts were deployed in the James Bulger trial. Indeed, in their evidence in court the child psychiatrists who interviewed the boys were not asked to offer any explanation for the boys' behaviour. Their evidence was confined to replying to the specific questions on the legal issue of *doli incapax* and whether they were suffering from an 'abnormality of mind' at the time of James Bulger's death and were capable of standing trial. Far from being called upon to identify and frame for public consumption 'the causes' of the boys conduct, psychiatry and psychology were reconstructed within law[26] and at the service of law, to enable the legal system to proceed as if the boys were fully responsible for their ter-

rible acts and to remove any remaining obstacles to their being convicted of James Bulger's murder.[27] After this had been achieved, it
was up to law, and not the behavioural or medical sciences, to interpret the events for society.[28]

It is also interesting to note that neither boy was offered any psychiatric treatment during the eight-month period while awaiting
trial, despite the psychiatric diagnosis that at least one of them was
suffering from 'post-traumatic stress disorder'. No doubt there were
good legal reasons for this denial of treatment in that such treatment with its inevitable rehearsal of past events might arguably have
contaminated the boys' memories and made them less reliable as
witnesses.[29] However, within the autopoietic framework, one might
also suggest that, once the event had been coded by the legal system
as one to which the criminal law applied, and the boys had been
charged with the crime, it was necessary, if confusion between those
functionally differentiated subsystems which we identified in
Chapter 1 were to be avoided, to delay any treatment until after the
trial. Within law one does not deal with potential criminals by
analysing their psyches and subjecting them to treatment. Such
treatment, if it comes at all, has to await the result of the trial.[30]

The search for causes

Once the Bulger affair had been coded as a legal issue the expectation was raised that the legal system's operations would result in
reassurances for society. This expectation was that, if found guilty,
the two boys would be removed from circulation for a very long
time; they would be safely 'behind bars'.[31] Once this had been
achieved, the risk to society's health came not from them personally,
but from the social evil(s) that had caused their corruption and
from the possibility that other corrupted children would repeat this
kind of unspeakable act. The trial judge speculatively identified one
of the evils as 'violent videos', but, as we have seen, outside the
courtroom the search for the evil at large within society ranged
much wider than that.

The question, 'Why were these meanings and not others privileged by society at a particular time?' always creates problems for
the theoretical framework of closed social systems theory. If it
could be known in advance what sense society would make of any
event, there would be no risk and uncertainty in the world. Political
parties, once elected, could govern forever, stock markets would

cease to exist and court trials would be unnecessary except as formalities and there would certainly be no place for any theory of autopoietic systems. Even for retrospective accounts, such as the one presented here, written with advantage of hindsight, to offer a definitive explanation for historical events is to assume presumptuously that only one correct version exists. Yet there may be as many causes to identify as there are possible interpretations of social events. Allan Levy, for example, in an article in the Tom Sargant Memorial Lecture,[32] saw in the Bulger trial and its aftermath 'the victimization of children' resulting from 'an increasingly reactionary approach in the criminal justice system' – a reaction which, he claims, is motivated by a politicization of law and order. Yvonne Roberts in *New Statesman and Society*, viewed the same events as evidence of a moral panic, which is what happens when society is undergoing 'profound social change'.[33] If, however, one abandons the impossible quest for definitive causes and turns more modestly to tracing the ways that meaning is produced, by and through a process of reconstruction and reinterpretation crosses the boundary between different social systems of communication, events such as the James Bulger murder, the trial of the two boys, and its aftermath come to be seen as matters of contingency rather than causality. One can never be certain why they occurred or if or when similar events will occur again. The communications of one system produced resonances or perturbations in another or others (be they social or psychic). Any explanation exists only as a retrospective account produced by an observer (or observing system) and as such has no authoritative claim for privilege over any other possible explanations. All that a theory which observes these observers may safely do is make its own observations available for deliberation.

JUSTICE AND WELFARE

The published accounts explaining the events following the brutal killing of James Bulger present the image of a society holding itself accountable for both the act and the actors. This image of self-recrimination involves, as we have shown, the projection of an archaic notion of 'evil' onto the two boys (and even onto Locke's *tabula rasa* of children in general) and hysterical demands for their punishment. If these accounts also represent vengeance and hatred of criminals and a call for their punishment as 'expressing and gratifying a healthy natural sentiment' advocated by the eminent

Victorian jurist, J. F. Stephen,[34] this does not necessarily indicate that nothing has changed since Stephen's day. Even if such 'healthy, natural sentiments' as 'deliberate anger and righteous disapprobation'[35] are still abundant today, the undoubted success of science has provided society with alternative forms of response to that of criminal justice. The difficulty for moralists such as Stephen is that these new 'scientific' forms did not recognize the existence of the evil which inspired such 'healthy natural sentiments', particularly where the 'criminal' is a child.

Nor is it possible to turn the clock back and see evil as the work of the devil or as God's temptation to man, as something external to society. Today, if evil finds its way into children, then the causes are to be found either within the child, in which case medical science reconstructs evil as mental illness or abnormality, whether genetic or caused by early experience; or within society, when social science is able to reconstitute evil as social factors correlating with violence, immoral and anti-social behaviour. In its search for scientifically sound explanations, therefore, science in its reconstruction of evil effectively annihilates the existence of evil. Put at its simplest, if medical and/or social science had been given the exclusive rights to make sense of the James Bulger murder, there would have been no talk of evil children.

Law in a certain sense is able to act a censor for such scientific amorality, confining it to a few exceptional cases. As we saw in the Bulger trial, psychiatry and psychology were reconstructed in law in the form of experts giving their opinion on the legal issues of *doli incapax* and mental impairment. In the evidence of the three experts, psychological science effectively disqualified itself from any right to present the killing as amenable to medical or scientific explanations.[36] Once these psychiatrists had handed over their written reports, these became in effect the property of law. Law was free to deal with the medico-scientific explanations they contained as it saw fit within the context of its own procedures, and in the Bulger case it saw fit to ignore them. Law cannot, however, control communications outside its own boundaries. Those meanings and attributions excluded by the legal system continue to exist outside its closed domain. In spite of the legal ruling that the boys were both sane and capable of responsibility for the deliberate act of murder, the search for scientific explanations for their behaviour and for the social circumstances which made such behaviour possible, continued both in journalistic writings and no doubt in the form of widespread, unrecorded psychological, sociological speculations as to the motives of Jon and Robert and as to the possible social factors to account for such an unlikely event.

While the threat of moral disorder in the unrestrained presence of evil within society may have been contained by the law's reconstitution of the evil as crime, the equally damaging prospect of unknown sociological, psychological or biological elements which could, if uncontrolled, lead to aberrant and dangerous behaviour in children, had not. Any claim to control through understanding scientifically the boys' conduct and the psychological and social factors which made such conduct possible carried with it the serious risk of failure or the equally serious risk of being left with multiple scientific understandings and no way of determining which one is scientifically 'correct'. Yet, paradoxically, it is precisely because the admission of uncertainty and, what is far worse, the irrefutable prospect of continuing uncertainty, would immediately condemn such explanations for crime to the scrap-heap of science, that it has been possible to reconstruct within the political system a scientific account of people's aberrant, irrational or anti-social behaviour, an account which reproduces scientific communications as part of *political programmes*. The fact that such accounts are impossible to prove or disprove *scientifically*, depending upon concepts which are themselves constructs of 'unscientific' communicative systems, allows them to thrive within the political arena. Seen in this light, the emergence in the last century and its rapid development within this century of 'welfare' as a *politically* acceptable alternative to Stephen's 'criminal justice' is not altogether surprising.[37]

In the United Kingdom the distinction between 'justice' and 'welfare' has been formalized into a political distinction characterizing until very recently the different approaches of the two main political parties towards the socially unacceptable behaviour of children. The Conservatives have favoured using criminal justice to condemn and punish juvenile crime, while the Labour Party has emphasized understanding underlying 'causes' and eradicating them either outside the courts or in problem-oriented family courts.[38] The one has seen the control of juvenile crime as a matter of individual and family discipline to be reinforced by the degradation and stigmatization of the offender; the other has looked to social workers and psychological experts to help resolve the underlying problems that have given rise to the child's behaviour. This symbiotic relationship and co-evolution[39] of politics, science and law around the issue of uncontrollable children was clearly visible from the Bulger case, which would have been dealt with outside the criminal law if the section of the Labour Government's Children and Young Persons Act, 1969, raising the age of criminal responsibility to 14, had been put into effect. A change of government and divisions within the Labour Party throughout the 1970s on the issue of juvenile offending effectively made it possible for two 10-year-old boys to be found guilty of murder.

Once the combined efforts of law, politics and science had made it possible for the evil of James Bulger's death to be classified as a crime, it was only to be expected that the political system would reconstruct the event in terms of its existing categories for dealing with crimes by juveniles, which reflected policy differences between government and opposition. Thus the Conservative Prime Minister, in a response to a parliamentary question on the murder of James Bulger, was able to refer to the failure of 'welfare approaches', adding that 'we should condemn more and understand less'. It was also to be expected that after the trial judge, during his sentencing speech, had honoured the court with his own psychological insight that 'exposure to violent videos may in part be an explanation',[40] the issue of the distribution of 'video nasties' would be taken up by some politicians in a way that left little doubt that these videos had been one of the real causes of James Bulger's death.[41] What was urgently needed, they argued, was effective legislation to regulate the distribution of violent videos to prevent them corrupting children by putting evil (and criminal) ideas into their heads.[42]

Science with law, welfare with justice

Within the environments of both law and science the choices available to make sense of James Bulger's killing by two 10-year-old boys take the form of clear mutually exclusive categories, which form the foundation for decisions. Either it is a legal issue or it is not. In the Bulger case the matter was resolved for law by the minimum age of 10 years for legal responsibility and by the evidence of the psychiatrists that it was not (for law) a medico-scientific issue. For science, it is either an issue to which scientific criteria for understanding may be applied or it is not. Within science the concepts of guilt or innocence, crime or no crime have no meaning. Either there is condemnation or there is understanding – two incompatible ways of categorizing and operating upon the phenomenon of children's. [43]

Reconstructed within politics, however, these first appear as stark choices between welfare *or* justice, but very soon merge as compromises, the integration of science-with-law, welfare-with-justice or justice-with-welfare. Even the Conservative Prime Minister talks in the relative terms of '*more* condemnation' and '*less* understanding'.

For those who operate at this level of converged systems there is blissful ignorance of the conceptual strains and stresses involved in such compromises. Gitta Sereny, for example, recommends 'combining the best elements of both' – the therapeutic treatment approach of the French model and the formal setting of the English criminal courts.[44] Allan Levy QC calls for '*more*, not *less* recognition' of 'the fact of childhood' within the criminal justice system and Stewart Asquith, Director of the Glasgow University Centre for the Study of the Child and Society, advocates 'a close working relationship between criminal and social policy'. He refers to the existing 'twin track approach' which characterizes Scottish and Continental European institutional approaches towards youth crime, whereby 'punishment and judicial proceedings are seen to be inappropriate for the majority of children', but appropriate for 'the minority of serious or persistent offenders'.[45]

The possibilities for interpretation now appear to become more complex. Instead of the straightforward binary choice between law or science, justice or welfare, punishment or treatment, the problem is how to establish the 'right balance' between the two. In this way risks of damaging children and society, either through over-harsh or over-formal measures or, alternatively, through responses which are insufficiently structuring or disciplining to the developing child, may apparently be minimized. In practice, of course, the choice between alternatives of law or science, justice or welfare, is not avoided but reproduced within the different institutions and practices which have developed through political compromises. From where, for example, do the criteria emerge that enable courts to decide what is a 'serious or persistent offender'? What determines whether an individual offender is more likely to alter his behaviour if punished than if given therapy or material assistance? The success of these institutions and practices in avoiding these hard questions by giving their operations the matter-of-fact appearance of rationality, with psychiatrists working alongside barristers and policemen, coordinating their activities with those of social workers, does not mean that choices have not been and are not being made, but rather that these distinctions have been banalized into everyday practices within these hybrid institutions to the point where the incompatibility of communicative systems, their system closure, no longer presents a problem. It is only when these operations are submitted to examination by external observations that inherent stresses and strains begin to appear as visible cracks in the structure.

At times when society believes itself to be in crisis the expectation that a simple moral solution does indeed exist may temporarily smother any alternative interpretations and block any communications which do not address the prevailing moral dilemma. At such times displays of unity and cooperation between communicative systems in producing a version of reality which both provokes anxiety and contains within it the means of relieving this anxiety, should not be mistaken for a suspension of the functioning of the operative closure of communicative systems. A cool retrospective examination will usually reveal that one system alone has been responsible for managing the disturbance, reconstructing others in ways which conform to its reassuring realities. For the violent killing of James Bulger this system, as we have seen, was law. Only after the legal system had defined with precision the nature of the 'evil' which confronted society was it possible for other systems to reconstruct the events within their own environments.

Moral crises of this kind are by their very nature of limited duration. Historically, it makes little sense to treat them, as some commentators have done, as denoting social revolutions, sudden and dramatic change of direction. Any changes in the ways that the world and events in that world are understood, take place over long periods and should not be confused with the spontaneous resonances of systems designed to relieve the irritating anxiety, respond to worrying perturbations, and provide reassurance that everything is under control. The rapid legal and political responses to the conviction of James Bulger's young murderers, in, for example, the short-lived abolition of the presumption of *doli incapax* for children between 10 and 14 by the High Court,[46] and the statutory measures passed by the British Parliament outlawing video nasties and implementing harsher punishments for children who commit crimes, did not represent, as some have suggested, sudden dramatic changes in the meaning of childhood and/or society's attitude towards children. Within social communications these changes in the conceptualization and understanding of children had been going on for some considerable time. Indeed, it could be argued that this heightened concern about children and their moral welfare will always exist as a continuous irritation, forcing social systems frequently to revise their reformulations of what children are and what childhood consists of and, in doing so, project their version of society's future. The media coverage of the James Bulger affair and its aftermath merely made these perennial concerns about children and childhood more widely visible by displaying them within the public arena.

Yet for an observer of the operations of society's closed systems the lesson to be learnt from the James Bulger affair is not that of the superiority of science over retributive law and a morality expressed through religious imagery. The many different speculative quests for the 'real causes' of the tragic killing of James Bulger – whether undertaken in the psychological development of his young killers, the material and emotional environment in which the two boys grew up, the relationship between their respective parents or the behaviour patterns of those adults who failed to intervene in James' abduction – all share a common objective. They seek to gain access to a truth, a certainty, that will offer the appealing prospect of reform and improvement and lead ultimately to solutions to the problems that they themselves have identified. Such 'scientific' endeavours are no more or less likely to succeed in their search than the hunt for the evil in our midst and the accusing finger pointed at ourselves for our past failures to recognize its existence. Both undertakings serve as a reassurance that something, at least, is being done and both construct in the present the prospect of a future society that is more predictable and more under control than that which exists. One should certainly not mock at these endeavours for, from a moral perspective, any possibility of a brighter future appears much more useful in the production of stable images of society and children in society than the kind of distanced sociological observation that is offered in this book. It hardly helps to reassure present anxieties over the future to take as one's starting point for an analysis of the killing of James an unlikely combination of economic, political, scientific, and legal events which began in the late eighteenth century and evolved eventually to give rise to such phenomena as people living in isolation or in small family units within massive conurbations, transported hither and thither by fast-moving machines, where relations between people are often characterized by distance, indifference or hostility; of the frequent separation of parents with young children, or of parents so demoralized, exhausted or so busy that they have little time or energy to devote to their children; of schools which confine children for a substantial part of their early lives and which some children do their best to avoid; of massive commercial shopping arcades, precincts and centres where these same children are able to spend the day stealing and mischief-making; of governments which have become the only source of food, clothing and housing for large numbers of people, and which themselves depend for their ability to provide these resources upon a global economic system; and so on *ad infinitum*.

NOTES

1 See, for example, Hall, 1978; Cohen, 1980; Hay, 1995.
2 See Chapter 1, pages 19–21.
3 See pages 13–19.
4 AIDS, for example, was in some religious communications designated an evil which God has inflicted on certain members of society as a punishment for their evil conduct. Scientific communications inform us, however, that it is simply a virus, to which moral attributions are not appropriate.
   Another example comes from a recent court decision made on 9 December 1994 when the law was able to define the abduction from hospital of a newly born baby as an act of desperation by a mentally disturbed woman and so not amenable to moral coding, despite the distress caused to the baby's parents (*The Guardian*, 10 December 1994).
5 The particular kind of paradox referred to, the paradox of the system's separation from its environment, is discussed in Chapter 3, pages 57–59. See also Luhmann (1989, p. 144) and King and Schütz (1994).
6 See Chapter 1, pages 26–28.
7 At first sight this analysis does not appear to work particularly well in those countries, such as Italy, where media comment on the crime and the accused is permitted before any finding of guilt. Such variations do not, however, detract from the main point that the matter is *sub judice* – under the authority of law – even if that authority grinds exceedingly slowly and some pre-trial press comment on the case is permitted. Even moral judgments in these situations have to recognize that authority.
8 Reported in *The Times*, 24 November 1993.
9 25 November 1993, p. 28.
10 The three evils identified as existing in 'the lexicon of crime' are 'metaphysical evil, the imperfection of all mankind; . . . physical evil, the suffering that humans cause each other; and . . . moral evil, the choice of vice over virtue'.
11 One wonders whether this *Times* leader writer reads novels or watches films. Fictional accounts of evil children are numerous. They include *The Exorcist, Lord of the Flies, The Omen, Damien – Omen II* and *Village of the Damned*. One could argue that children representing the

paradox of evil–innocence is one which is pervasive in contemporary culture.

12 *The Times*, 25 November 1993.
13 *ibid.*
14 28 November 1993, p. 3.
15 See Luhmann (1992)
16 Niklas Luhmann writes:

> More and more states – whether existing or aspired to – are seen as being consequent to decisions, i.e. are attributed to decisions. Much is due to the dual intervention of the more pervasive technological development and more pronounced individualization of entities and processes formerly regarded as constituting Nature.
>
> (Luhmann, 1993, p. 46)

17 This is what Luhmann refers to as *deparadoxification*, that is, the concealment of the self-referential nature of society's interpretative systems, the fact that their authority is self-imposed and self-perpetuated.
18 Literally, incapable of guile or deceit
19 The Divisional Court case of *C.* v. *DPP* [1994] Crim. LR subsequently decided that the presumption of innocence is no longer part of English criminal law. This decision, however, was reversed on appeal.
20 The comparable age in France is 13. See J. Bourquin (1994) 'The James Bulger Case Through the Eyes of the French Press', *Social Work in Europe',* 1(1): p. 42. The age of criminal responsibility in other European countries ranges from 18 in Belgium, Romania and Lithuania to 7 in Switzerland and Ireland. In Scandinavian countries it is 15 (see Dunkel, 'Legal Differences in Juvenile Criminology in Europe' in T. Booth (ed.) *Juvenile Justice in the New Europe*, Social Services Monograph: Research in Practice. Allan Levy QC, in an article published by *Justice* 'castigated the Government for not implementing legislation passed by Parliament in 1969 raising the age of criminal responsibility to 14'. *The Guardian*, 25 November 1994.
21 See Smith (1994) and Sereny (1994).
22 We need look no further than the problems that psychology has in making unequivocal statements about what is good or bad for children. The controversies surrounding the advantages and disadvantages for children of separated parents to retain a regular contact with the non-residential parent and the arguments over whether conflict between, or the separation of, parents causes the greater harm to the child are but two current examples of the difficulties of converting psychological findings into moral (or legal) principles.
23 See, for example, almost any edition of the *Newsletter of the Criminological and Legal Division of the British Psychological Society.*
24 See the M'Naghton criteria for the defence of insanity.
25 See Homicide Act, 1957 Section 2(1) criteria for the defence of diminished responsibility.
26 This construction within the legal system of psychology-within-law is discussed in detail in King and Piper (1995).
27 Perhaps the closest that anyone involved in the trial came to a psycho-

logical explanation came not from any 'psy' expert, but from the barrister who defended Robert Thompson, in his closing speech to the jury.

> These boys were saddled by their own mischief with a little toddler who must have been tired out, as they were themselves. They had been hanging around the shops at the Strand since school time in the morning, walking with a toddler all that way, not knowing what to do with him, unable to abandon him or foist him off on a grown-up, and not having the courage to take him into a police station where they had taken him because they might have been afraid that they would be in trouble. This a far more likely scenario than the planned evil put forward by the Crown.

28 Neither the reports of the three psychiatrists who examined the boys nor the assessment of Jon by a clinical psychologist were referred to during the trial. They were not even mentioned by Judge Morland when he came to pass sentence.
29 In the event neither of them was called by the defence to give evidence.
30 One is reminded of the Sutcliffe (Yorkshire Ripper) case when, a few months after the defence of insanity was rejected by the jury, Sutcliffe was transferred from prison to a secure mental hospital suffering from a psychotic illness.
31 The trial judge recommended that they should not be released for eight years minimum. This was increased by the Lord Chief Justice to ten years and finally by the Home Secretary, in response to a petition submitted by supporters of the Bulger family demanding that the boys should never be released, to fifteen years. This final decision is at present being challenged in the European Court for Human Rights, having been criticized by the Commission for its contravention of the European Convention.
32 Reproduced in a shortened version in *The Guardian*, 29 November 1994.
33 'Teaching Children to be Bad', 3 December 1993, pp. 14–15.
34 (1883) p. 82. See Smith (1988, pp. 56–60).
35 *ibid.*
36 There was no redress, for example, against the judge's decision not to refer to the medical evidence in his decision as to the appropriate length of time that the boys should remain in detention.
37 See generally Garland (1988). For an account of the emergence of the concept of 'welfare' in relation to juvenile offenders and the parameters of the justice versus welfare debate, see Chapter 1 of King and Piper (1995, note 38).
38 See, for example, the Labour Government's White Papers in the 1960s, *The Child, the Family and the Young Offender* and *Children in Trouble*. The 'new realism' introduced by Tony Blair, the present leader of the opposition Labour Party, when he was Shadow Home Secretary, reduced the difference between the policies of the parties, but never-

theless retained 'understanding the causes of crime' as an important element in the party's policy.

39 In Luhmann's terms, *structural coupling*.

40 See Smith *op. cit.* at p. 227. As Smith points out, 'there had been no mention in evidence of any videos', but only rumours that the boys may have watched *Child Play 3*. Yet even if they had seen this film, there is apparently little or nothing in the film to connect it to the killing of James Bulger.

41 A measure was introduced by the government into Part VII of the Criminal Justice and Public Order Act, 1994 which provided for stricter censorship of videos than is available for films shown publicly.

42 As a direct result of this concern over the effects of videos on children's behaviour, the Criminal Justice and Public Order Act, which received royal assent in November 1994, contains provision for stricter censorship over videos available to the public.

43 This is not to suggest that condemnation and punishment cannot themselves become items for scientific investigation or that the activities of science cannot themselves become the subject of legal disputes.

44 Sereny (1994, note 23, p. 11).

45 Asquith (1996).

46 See note 19, above.

Chapter 6

Real and imagined communities and families

COMMUNITISM AND FAMILIALISM

In 1991 a book entitled, *Imagined Communities*, appeared (Anderson, 1991) in which the author traces the origin and global spread of nationalism from Western countries to developing nations. This chapter by way of contrast considers what at first sight appears to be a reversal in the normal pattern of globalization by reflecting upon the attempt to reform decision making procedures concerning children and young people transporting 'community' and 'family' from their assumed roots in custom and tradition to the complex urban sprawl of post-industrial cities – from the romanticized jungle to the concrete jungle.

The terms, 'communitism' and 'familialism', which I shall be using, need some explaining. In the first place communitism should not be confused with 'communism' and 'communitarianism', which for political scientists denote very clear and distinctive approaches to the organization of society, invoking the notion of perfection, or at least the best of all possible worlds. Unlike communitarianism, communism, socialism, feminism, liberalism and many other utopian 'isms', communitism is a faintly disparaging term designed to put down those romantic people who claim that they have the answer to the problems of modern society and that this answer lies in the general panacea of returning to those forms of life and morality which, they claim, existed in the good old times, before society grew in size and complexity and before these traditional forms were destroyed by another set of 'isms', this time non-utopian, which could include colonialism, capitalism, consumerism and nationalism.

Communitists and familialists then have much in common.

Communitists see the social world as consisting of communities which are always good things to be preserved and protected wherever they can be found. Where they do not exist, they should, wherever possible, be constructed, resurrected and recreated. Familialism highlights families as having all the positive attributes of small-scale communities, but with the additional advantage of being fairly easy to identify and define, for families exist through the medium of blood ties, which in the world inhabited by familialists, automatically forge bonds of affection and responsibility between members. Generally these bonds tend to be seen as even stronger than those which bind unrelated members of a community.

Both communitism and familialism tell us that the traditional values are best and that only by returning to them will we be able to halt the evils of bureaucracy, tyranny by experts, bureaucratic interference, the police state, etc. It is these values which will stop the rot and bring society back to its senses. Such beliefs, however, must not be dismissed lightly; they demand the careful consideration that we shall be giving to them after a brief account of recent events which have linked the ideals of communitism and familialism with decisions concerning children.

THE ROOTS OF FAMILY GROUP CONFERENCES

Our story starts in New Zealand where, according to W. R. Atkin, writing in the *Journal of Family Law*, after decades of exploitation and deprivation the Maori people, 'experienced a gradual awakening of their spirituality, their influence and their culture . . .' (Atkin, 1988–1989, p. 231). He goes on to explain that:

> [I]n traditional Maori terms, the important concepts for personal relationships are *whanau*, the *hapu*, and the *iwi*. A rough translation which fails to do justice to these words, is, respectively, 'extended family', 'sub-tribe', and 'tribe'. . . . The *whanau* is the basic family unit from which the parent–child relationship develops . . . the responsibility for bringing up children does not rest solely with the birth parents, but is shared by adult relatives. The *hapu* will have between one hundred and one thousand members, all having common ancestors. The *iwi* is a much larger kinship linkage where members share a common ancestor.
>
> (Atkin, 1988–1989, pp. 231–232)

The reason why this brief excursion into traditional Maori society is necessary is that in 1987 a Report of a Working Party on the issues of child protection and juvenile crime (Department of Social Welfare, 1987) gave official government recognition to the importance of the *whanau, hapu* and *iwi* in the care and upbringing of children and, in doing so, questioned the cultural appropriateness of 'the paramountcy principle', that legacy from the English legal system, which made the child's welfare paramount in any legal decision and, it was argued, allowed *Pakeha* (Colonial) justice to impose its values upon indigenous families in determinations of what was best for the child. The Working Party recommended replacing this principle by requiring any court exercising powers under the new act

> in the first instance [to] address the rights and needs of a child or young person *in the context of their family of belonging – whanau, hapu or iwi, family group* and the potential within such groupings to effect such changes as may be necessary to promote and preserve the well-being of their children and young people.
> (Department of Social Welfare, 1987, p. 27, emphasis added)

What eventually emerged from this search for a 'culturally sensitive' and 'culturally appropriate' system of justice was the *family group conference*. This is an alternative and very different forum for decision making to courts of law. In family group conferences people from the child's 'family' or 'community' discuss the child's situation (often in the presence of the child) and are expected to arrive at some solution which, in the case of young offenders, will both bring the children or young people to accept responsibility for their misbehaviour and involve the victim in devising some appropriate punishment or compensation. In child abuse cases, it will protect the child and promote its welfare.

The concept of 'conferences' has sparked off intense interest among law reformers throughout all those post-industrial countries which still use courts of law as the principal forum for decision making in child protection and juvenile crime.[1] The 1989 New Zealand model has been adapted, either in its original or a modified form, in several places in Australia and the original child protection version duplicated by the Family Rights Group in England as a voluntary alternative to court decision making. Family group conference projects have also been started in Newfoundland and British Columbia. It has incidentally also succeeded in expanding the English language, turning 'conference' into a verb, so that it is now possible to talk of 'conferencing' a child or a family, or of a case having been 'conferenced'.

It is not the intention at this point to discuss the detailed procedures of the conference system, but rather to raise certain queries concerning the claim made by those promoting the conference system as an effective alternative to the courts both in criminal and child protection cases, that it makes excellent sense to use the concepts 'community' and 'family' as units for decision making in the modern world. Of course, it is easy to criticize the introduction of family group conferences in areas or countries which are not blessed with the equivalent of the Maori *whanau* or *hapu*. Professor Michael Freeman, for example writes that the South Australian Family Group Meeting concept is 'essentially flawed', as '[t]he *whanau* has no counterpart in South Australia.' (Freeman, 1994). But as Atkin points out, in its traditional form the *whanau* and *whanautatanga* (kinship feeling) has by now lost all or much of its power for Maoris in New Zealand. Many of them have married non-Maoris. Many have now migrated from their traditional lands to the big cities and suburbs. 'In some places' he remarks 'urban *whanau* have been established, but they are new and do not necessarily depend upon blood ties' (Atkin, 1988–1989, p. 232). The flawlessness or perfection of the conference concept, therefore, does not depend upon the verifiable existence of an ongoing family, child-caring, child-sharing cooperative, but on something rather different – the universal appeal of the idealized notions of 'family' and 'community'.

THE MARKETING OF FAMILY GROUP CONFERENCES

It goes without saying that there is much more going on here than a 'back to basics' appeal to family and community values. One only has to read the powerful and sophisticated arguments in John Braithwaite's publicity material extolling the benefits of replacing juvenile courts with conferencing, to realize that buying into family group conferences gives you much more than just 'cultural appropriateness'. What it is able to offer is 'a form of communitarianism' and 'a communitarian process' (Braithwaite, 1992, p. 40), 'community accountability' (Braithwaite, 1994, p. 199), 'a community accountability model' (*ibid.*, p. 206) 'citizen ceremonies of reintegrative shaming' and 'the giving back of conflicts to people (Braithwaite, 1992, p. 37, Braithwaite, 1993, Braithwaite and Petit, 1990). According to Braithwaite, 'A successful conference is one where the offenders are brought to experience remorse for the effects of their crimes and to understand that they can count on the continuing support, love and respect of their families and friends' (Braithwaite, 1992, p. 37).

He goes on to argue that in any event, 'cultural appropriateness' in the narrow sense of Aboriginal values, may not be what is required even for the effective shaming, support and reintegration of young Aboriginals, for

> in an urban setting the Aboriginal elders will not necessarily be people the young Aboriginal will know or respect. The idea of a family group conference is to assemble in the room the particular Aboriginal people who care about a particular Aboriginal young person. It mobilizes a community process on both the victim and the offender side . . . *it is a form of communitarianism that can and does work in large multicultural cities.*
>
> (Braithwaite, 1992, p. 37, emphasis added)

It is clear, therefore, from Braithwaite's various accounts that 'family' does not necessarily mean a group of blood relations and community need not have its Shorter Oxford Dictionary meaning of 'a body of people organized into a political, municipal or social unity'. Instead these terms may be given meanings which allow Braithwaite and his fellow supporters of family group conferences to include a wide variety of people, whose common feature is a feeling of concern for the child or young person – 'the offender and supporters of the offender (usually the nuclear family . . . sometimes neighbours, counsellors, even a teacher or football coach)' (Braithwaite and Mugford, 1994). In the case of juvenile offenders it will also involve the victim of the crime (and supporters of the victim, usually from the nuclear family), those people, in other words, who claim to have been harmed by the offender's behaviour.

In their many writings on the subject Braithwaite and his colleagues[2] extol the virtues of family group conferences as heralding a major policy change away from state control towards 'republicanism' and 'communitarianism', and denounce the courts and the criminal justice process as offering only a stigmatizing with entirely negative effects for the young offender, while doing little or nothing to solve society's major problem of juvenile crime. The ultimate proof of the value of 'conferencing', they argue, is whether it works in practice. This, they argue, is entirely a matter for empirical research and, according to them, all the evidence so far indicates that it is working well.

These are powerful arguments. They are also very difficult to counter, as critics of 'conferencing' experienced at a meeting held at the Australian Institute of Criminology in Canberra in 1994. Here criticisms that conferences were not 'working as well' as Braithwaite and his critics had maintained, were met with the response that any failures could be attributed to 'conference malpractice' (Braithwaite, 1994, p. 199). There was good conferencing and there was 'terrible conferencing' just as there are 'some terrible juvenile court proceedings and terrible police cautions' (*ibid.*). The task ahead was to ensure that all conferences were 'good'. The worth of conferences, according to Braithwaite, can be assessed on 'a number of evaluative dimensions', not by failures in performance, but by their 'good and bad effects' (*ibid.*). In other words, the proof of the pudding is in the eating. If such matters as re-offending rates, victim satisfaction and offenders' completion rates of the punishment assigned to them showed an improvement over the processes of conventional juvenile justice, there was ample justification for claiming that conferencing was a better solution than courts and police cautions.

Nevertheless, several of the delegates to the Canberra meeting were left with the uneasy feeling that something was seriously wrong with a process of decision making which seeks its credentials in democratized social control, but (in the case of the Australian scheme) is organized and supervised by the police (Sandor, 1994); which claims its roots in community values and yet fails 'to address the major questions of unemployment, inadequate schools and institutional racism' (Polk, 1994); and, furthermore, which offers to improve the life-chances of children and young people and yet reinforces the stigmatizing notion that they are always to blame for their offending behaviour (White, 1994). These criticisms, however, tend to rely upon sets of ideological beliefs about the nature of society and the motives of individuals and operations of social institutions, which are open to the same kind of challenge that the critics direct against the claims of Braithwaite and his colleagues. Those who argue that they are better than others at appreciating and promoting justice or fairness and at recognizing and condemning state coercion and abuse of power, are obliged to rely upon some notion of the truth which sees their beliefs about society and individuals as superior to the beliefs of others. In practice these conflicting claims between sets of belief cannot be resolved by scientific criteria or empirical proof, since they represent, not theories competing to explain the causes of phenomena, but different forms of political ideology. The choice of 'causes' for the phenomenon of juvenile crime – itself a social construction – will depend upon the political convictions of the observer and there is no scientific way of proving or disproving these convictions. Put in the terms of autopoietic system theory, described in Chapter 1, juvenile crime cannot be explained scientifically but, as we shall examine later, it may operate as a politically-inspired irritant for science, provoking within science attempts to reduce through theorizing and empirical testing the relationships between such crime and other factors, such as, in this case, different forms of decision making. These reductions, it must be emphasized can never become 'scientific knowledge' about the causes of crime, first because the concept of 'crime' is a social construct and cannot be defined in hard scientific terms, and second, because any attempt to identify and test the causes of crime will inevitably be selective in what it recognizes as possible causal factors or possible interrelationships between factors.

This is something which Braithwaite is wise enough to recognize and which his critics do not. Rather than entering into the battle about whose ideology is superior he simply states what he claims to be the philosophical pedigree of his approach and then plays the 'scientific' card to his advantage, turning the table on his critics by claiming that science and not politics can tell us whether family group conferences are working well or not. Of course, for Braithwaite science has a particular meaning, which involves using certain criteria in order to test empirically that family group conferences 'work'. These criteria of success do not depend on how well the process conforms with those highly contested notions of justice, equality, fairness, freedom, coercion, use and abuse of power, etc., but upon 'a number of evaluative dimensions' which, as we have seen, will reveal to us 'their good and bad effects' (Braithwaite, 1994, p.199).

In the place of irreconcilable differences between lofty ideals we are left with the mundane, practical empiricist's solution of 'if it works, according to my criteria, then it works'. The corollary of this seems to be that, if it does work and can be 'proved' to work, the theoretical principles on which the practical solutions are based must be right. In this way Braithwaite is able to compare the contested claims of different political ideologies in ways that make it appear that they are amenable to scientific testing. More specifically, if family group conferences appear, according to his empirical data, to 'work' by producing 'good effects' for the offender and the victim, the superiority of his self-styled communitarianism and republicanism over other forms of political organization, would, on Braithwaite's terms be confirmed.

One of the stated purposes of this book is to observe claims that it is possible to construct and regulate a world that will be better for children in some absolute sense. This act of observation has in its sights both the 'practical knowledge' of legal, political, social work and child welfare practitioners and equally those theories, principles and formulae which have in mind some utopian world where children are relieved of all suffering and protected against harms. Braithwaite's account of family group conferences and their apparent success would seem then to challenge the role of the observer taken throughout this book. Here, it seems, in family group conferences is a practical device built upon the firm foundations of objective reality and, according to its promoters, readily amenable to scientific evaluation of its ability to improve not only the decision making process, but also children's lives. What is more, this device is, it is claimed, underpinned by political theory and sustained by well-tried and tested tribal customs. It apparently transfers power from the hands of faceless state officials to the family and the community. It controls the undesirable behaviour of children and adults, not through punitive and coercive methods (which do more harm than good), but through the beneficial processes of shaming and integration.

If the object of this book had been to assess scientifically the effectiveness, practicality, and value of schemes and projects designed to improve the lives of children, we would have been obliged at this stage to lock into the debate that engages Braithwaite and his critics. This, however, is not its object. What it seeks to do rather is to view designs for the future well-being of children from a vantage point where these designs are neither approved of nor challenged directly, but simply observed as the construction of a reality, not the only reality. This should not be seen as avoidance of the question 'What is good for children?', but as a challenge to the very idea that such a question has any meaning except within the constructed world of social communication systems. Far from arguing for the superiority of one set of ideological values over another or offering absolute truths about children and their needs, the exercise undertaken by this book places values and truths within closed conceptual frameworks – social systems – and proposes that the debates about what is good or bad for children makes sense only within the context of these systems (Stainton Rogers, 1992).

In using one theory to observe projects which emerge from very different ways of seeing society and 'its problems', there is, of course, the risk that the reader will be left in a postmodernist limbo of confusion and relativism. Yet this is only a problem if one sees the quest for right and wrong answers as the ultimate or only legitimate objective. Of course, there is no one or nothing (not even science) to tell us which theory or ideology is the right one and which the wrong one. Observations which seek to locate the project within the broad framework of a structured system of continually-evolving meaning called 'society' (see pages 26–28) may be able to throw some light on those parts of the system which are obscured by the necessarily blinkered and partial vision of specific projects and the ways of seeing the world that they represent. These kinds of observation may be able to reveal what the project or theory cannot see. But this is not all; they may also be able to observe the critical observers of the project or theory and to see that they themselves were operating within a limited framework where only a part of the whole is visible. To observe, for example, John Braithwaite's account of family group conferences, should not oblige the observer to join the ranks of the critics at the Canberra conference in order to demonstrate that Braithwaite's ideas are wrong in some absolute sense and that family group conferences are likely to do more harm than good to children and young people. Even to engage in such an exercise forces the observer to accept the assumptions that absolute right and absolute wrong are able to exist conceptually and that it is possible to prove empirically in an unequivocal manner what harms and what benefits children and young people.

May it not also be a useful exercise to locate the family group conference within a shifting ephemeral world of communications where delusions have to represent reality and where assurance for the future is seen as depending upon the ability to make sense of and control the present? What might evolve from such an exercise?

SOCIAL PROBLEMS AND THEIR RESOLUTION

Simply to see family group conferences as a solution to a problem, or rather, as a solution to several problems, does not take sociological observation very far, since social problems have no more claim to an authentic objectivity than the solutions conceived for their resolution. Problems are not things; they are constructions of states of affairs and events which give rise to anxieties and the call for solutions (Spector and Kitsuse, 1977; Manning, 1985). These constructions, even where they relate exclusively to products of nature, such as earthquakes or droughts, take the form of situations which are perceived as giving rise to risks which are both assessable and, up to a point, controllable (Beck, 1992; Luhmann, 1993, p. 35). The social construction of social problems which created the apparent need for family group conferences starts, not with families or communities, but with the conduct of young people who commit crimes and parents who abuse and neglect their children. Both of these events are of course socially defined, as the concepts of crime, abuse and neglect are interpretations of behaviour and, what is more, interpretations which permit the development of further interpretations, such as the identification of risks of children engaging in crime or of becoming victims of child abuse and neglect, as well as the risks to the future stability of society through, for example, the damage that crime and child abuse supposedly create for the family and the community.

At the level of social communications, that is, communication within and between social systems, these collective anxieties, constructed as social problems, exist as irritants to systems, generating the need for a response – but always in a form that has meaning within the responding system. The legal system, therefore, will respond to social problems with legal communications, the political system with political communications, science with scientific communications and so on. Such responses are quite independent of the effects on and reactions of individuals or conscious systems.

It needs to be emphasized at this point that we are dealing here with communications and not with structures which have any physical form. These structures exist only as systems which recognize communications as belonging or not belonging to that system. The legal, scientific, and political systems in this diagram exist only as ways of making sense of social events including communications from other systems. We start with the statement that juvenile crime has increased – a communication made possible by society's already existing distinction of behaviour into criminal/not criminal and by the measures developed within science for identifying increases and decreases in crime. This 'problem', amplified by the press and broadcasting media, becomes an irritant for politics. It may, for example, be interpreted as an indication that government is failing to deal effectively with risks to the safety of vulnerable people or their possessions. This demands a response from the government of the day – new laws or increased spending on the police or on surveillance, or a programme of activities to occupy the time and energy of young people. This response will have implications for other social function systems. Law, for example, may be faced with new legal issues concerning the criminal responsibility of children, between behaviour which is unlawful and lawful (even if immoral – see Chapter 5). The increase in the costs of financing the legal system will have implications for economics – not only directly in terms of its demands on the budget, but also perhaps indirectly, if large numbers of the most gifted graduates choose to become lawyers and specialize in representing or prosecuting young people in the juvenile courts, rather than joining industry and producing wealth for the country. The response of economics to this irritant may well be to propose a more cost-effective system which places less value on the protection of individual rights than on the efficient processing of cases through the courts.

The same process of problem construction and risk-identification, followed by solution-responses generated by social communication systems may be traced for 'child abuse', although in this case it is the welfare of children and the health or normality of family relationships rather than 'the protection of society' which become the primary targets of system communications. In both cases, juvenile crime and child abuse, each solution-providing system is able to see only part of what is recognized by society as 'the problem'. The solutions offered, therefore, can be only partial solutions – not in the sense that any psychotherapeutic or social policy solution requires proper funding or the motivation of the deviant parents or children to change their ways, but rather because each system can see only what it can see and understand only what it can make sense of. Law then may well be able to make perfect sense of juvenile crime as a problem for law, whenever a criminal case involving a child or young person is presented to the courts, but it is quite unable to produce anything other than legal communications by way of response. The making of a probation order, for example, is no guarantee that the supervision provided by an over-stretched probation service will result in that young person turning away from his or her criminal activities, and no form of legal wording in the order is going to improve the chances of this happening. Similarly, there can be no certainty, or even probability, that an order removing a child from its abusive family will not result in that child's future welfare being damaged (whether or not society labels it, 'abuse') in a foster family or children's home. In other words, the success or failure of the legal communication in achieving its objective of contributing to the solution of social problems depends on matters outside the control of law. The same is true of scientific or therapeutic solutions which may easily be thwarted by legal interference, such as the confidentiality/secrecy, stresses or conflicts generated by an impending or recent court hearing (King and Trowell, 1992), the withdrawal of funding from therapeutic programmes, or even chance happenings, such as accidents, illness or bumping into an old friend in the street. In the case of many social problems, they are quite simply beyond control, if control means putting into effect measures which are certain to solve or relieve the problem.

A sceptical observer might wish here to draw the distinction between control and the illusion of control which may be seen as characterizing social communications, but the interdependency of social systems forbids such a distinction ever entering these communications, for recognizing an illusion in one system can only cast doubt on the certainties of another or others. To question the legal system's image of itself as playing an essential part in the control of crime or the protection of children is also to question the legitimacy of all those therapeutic and social welfare services which depend upon the continuing production of legal decisions. It is far preferable to revert to Braithwaite's distinction working/not working, for there is always contained within the negative side of the distinction the possibility of further distinctions, which will allow the observer to analyse what precisely is 'not working' and why; and with these distinctions the probability that solutions will be found to transform the process, to 'turn it round', so that, at least on the criteria by which it was at one time held not to be working, it now is seen to work. Of course, this does not prevent new distinctions giving rise to new criteria of 'working', which may well result in aspects of the newly reformed process finding themselves once again on the negative side of the working/not working distinction.

THE POLITICS OF 'COMMUNITY' AND 'FAMILY'

It is not hard to understand how the partial blindness of social communicative systems may be interpreted as ignorance, indifference or, in the worst cases, as stubborn refusal to recognize what to the observer is painfully obvious. The tendency today for people to be divided into racial, ethnic, and cultural groups as well as into the more traditional class, caste, age, gender and religious divisions, and for certain of these identities to transform themselves into political movements (Calhoun, 1994) in a largely unpredictable and haphazard manner may cause enormous difficulties for those systems on whose communications the continuing business of 'making society work' depends. Accusations of injustice, inequality, prejudice, or discrimination seem at times to overwhelm the 'normal operations' of these function systems. This may apply equally to the courts as to therapeutic remedies for relieving personal and family crises. Both are now suspected of disregarding or, even worse, of perpetuating those inequalities and injustices which underlie the marital conflict or mistreatment of children, reducing these issues of identity politics to legal arguments or psychological analyses.

The danger for the autonomy of society's function systems, law, science, economics, politics, etc., and so for society, is that of dedifferentiation – the point where systems lose their distinctive identity, their closure. The irritant of identity politics may be so pervasive, therefore, that legal, scientific, economic, educational communications abandon their self-referential operations and come to rely instead upon validations derived from one particular group which succeeds in imposing its definition of injustice and inequality. In this situation what is presented as politically necessary in order to redress past injustices and inequalities becomes accepted by society as lawful, scientifically truthful, profitable, educational, etc. This is not to suggest that society should deny any responsibility for redressing past wrongs, but rather that the entry within the function systems of modern society of distinctions based *entirely* upon these concerns for redress may have serious consequences for the operation of these systems. In the worst scenario, it may result in the gradual merging of these systems so that law, science, economics and politics are all engaged to one end – that of upholding and sustaining the rights, powers and privileges claimed by groups and substituting distinctions based upon notions of personal identity for those generated by the systems' internal operations.

The emergence of organizational forms based upon the idealized groupings or classifications of people may be seen as one way of avoiding this danger. Indeed, the attractiveness of family and community decision making and the like is their apparent neutrality in the warfare between one group identity and another. Families, almost by definition, are not exclusively men or women. As 'families' pure and simple they have no racial, ethnic or cultural identity which requires to be protected against or privileged over other such identities. Instead the family is presented as an autonomous unit, a closed system with the potential to develop its own self-referential existence. The same is true of 'communities'. These are represented either as being ethnically or culturally homogenous or undifferentiated, as in 'the Maori community' or 'the Islamic community' or as including a plurality of cultures and ethnic groups (and, of course, both genders) – 'the community' – in such a way that any differences of identity that do exist are subsumed into the undifferentiated whole and so relieved of their importance.

Family mediation is one of these new organizational forms. Here any decisions concerning future relations between members of a divorcing family enter society as 'family decisions'. The family thus becomes a black box into which observers are unable to peer. The decision or the resolution of the problem emerges as a family communication, but one which may have lasting consequences for the legal, economic and emotional future of parents and children, while, at the same time, relieving the courts of the risks involved in threading their way through a minefield of emotional turmoil and fractured identities.

Of course, such 'family decisions' may reflect structural inequalities which exist within families, both between men and women and between adults and children.[3] Similarly, questions of what is good or bad for children are left to parental negotiations, which may be influenced by subtle persuasion from mediators (Piper, 1993) or by medico-scientific or 'common sense' notions of child welfare. As it is, communications within the black box of the family remain hidden from the social gaze. They enter the level of social communications only as 'agreements' ready to be transformed into legal orders or decisions concerning home, financial support and education.[4]

The family group conference, as we have seen, is a form which combines or merges both notions, family and community, in ways which make it appear that the apparently divisive, distant and alienating processes of decision making about children and young people associated with formal courts of law may be avoided by bringing people together as a 'family' and/or 'community'. This new model of decision making is presented as being outside the formal legal system and, for that matter, any other of modern society's formal practices for coping with family problems, such as child psychiatry or family therapy.

In order to understand the nature of the social meanings that both enter these new forms and are being generated by them, we need to separate procedures from the structure of the communicative process. Simply to change the procedures which lead to legal decisions does not change their nature as legal decisions. Similarly, removing this process from a formal court building and situating it in the living room of a suburban home does not in itself make the decision any less legal. For autopoietic systems theorists, the essence of systems is not their physical environment, their procedures or even the particular characteristics of the people who operate them, but their distinctive communications. It is, for example, the distinctive nature of legal communications, their representation of the world in terms of lawfulness and unlawfulness, which allows them to be recognized as law both by the legal system and by other functional subsystems, such as politics or economics.

Conversely, if, and only if, the communications produced by family group conferences are recognized by society as legal communications, would it be proper to describe this new process as part of the legal system. In a similar manner, if and only if these communications were recognized as saying something meaningful about the physical or psychological well-being of the child could they be recognized as health or child-welfare communications. A court order that a father should not see his child, because of the danger of beatings, would have meaning both within law and child welfare. It could be judged both according to legal criteria – did the court exceed its powers and was there sufficient evidence presented for the court to reach the conclusion that the child would be in danger? – or according to the medico-scientific criteria of child welfare – in what ways are the beatings likely to harm the child, both physically and psychologically, and is this harm likely to exceed the harm caused by the lengthy absence of the father from the child's life? Knowing precisely how researchers propose to evaluate the decisions of family group conferences will, therefore, give us a strong indication of their meaning for the researcher, and of the social function system which is responsible for attributing this meaning.

THE SHADOW OF THE LAW

Let us examine first the family group conference as an alternative to the formal juvenile justice system which tries and sentences young offenders, by observing what was seen by researchers to occur in two case studies from a conferencing project in Wagga Wagga in the state of Victoria, Australia.[5] This is what the researchers reported in the first case:

Background

Following an early morning party, two 17-year-old and two 18-year-old-male offenders drove around Wagga Wagga throwing stones and other debris from the vehicle. They broke windows on five motor vehicles and a window at a local primary school. Damage was approximately $1,400.

Police intervention

Police received information from a friend of one of the offenders about two months after the incident. The offenders were interviewed, and initially, in view of the level of damage and the age of the offenders, police intended to place the matter before the court. However, it was decided that the case should be resolved by conference.

Cautioning process

The cautioning conference involved the following people:

- four offenders, parents, brothers, sisters, uncles and aunts;
- five victims, relations or friends;
- the reporting police officer;
- the sergeant as the cautioning officer.

The offenders gave a version of what had taken place. Each had difficulty in actually relating their version because of what had been described by their families as 'senseless acts'. Each victim told how this had affected them and their families. One victim (a young university student) explained that because he had no money, he had to contact his brother who paid to have the front screen on the vehicle replaced. He said that he was repaying his brother $10 each fortnight. Another victim explained that he spent two days consoling young schoolchildren and their teacher about the broken window.

When the conference participants were talking about restitution, the offenders volunteered full compensation and suggested that they undertake at least eighty hours community work. One victim believed that this was excessive. Another reminded them that they would shortly be undertaking their Higher School Certificate so time spent doing community work needed to be realistic.

Outcomes

- Each offender publicly apologized to the victim;
- the victims were satisfied with being involved and asked each offender to put this behind them;
- each offender agreed to pay his share of compensation and do forty hours community work;
- each offender publicly apologized to his own family;
- all families expressed dismay at what had taken place, but indicated their support for the offender, although they felt some trust needed to be restored.

What is immediately apparent from this case history is that the decision that emerged was not that of a family or community conference in the usual sense of these terms, but resulted rather from discussions and negotiations between the offenders and some of their family members, and the victims and some of their relations and friends. Not only was the discussion presided over by a police officer, but it was the police who had decided to hold a 'conference' in the first place. Furthermore, the way in which the participants were defined either as offenders and their relations, or victims and their relations and friends places the 'conference' firmly in the framework of the criminal law. It is not 'the community' which has come together to decide what should be done about the damage caused by four rowdy young men, but the police that have labelled the matter an offence and brought together 'offenders' and 'victims' to discuss how 'the offence' should be dealt with. The conference did not have the power to decide, for example, that parties should end by midnight or that no alcoholic drinks should be available to those under 20 years old. Nor was it expected to examine the backgrounds of each offender in the search for social or psychological factors which might have caused them to behave in such a way. What was available to them were similar powers to those of a court of law, namely, dealing with the matter in an individualized way as a crime and punishing those who had admitted committing the crime.

Apart from the obvious differences in procedures, what made the conference different from a court was the way that it was judged by the police and by the observer writing up the case study. These comments appear under the heading:

Issues

- The conference appeared to be a more appropriate option than court;
- victims contributed in a very positive way, which provided the offenders and their families with a good platform to resolve issues of trust, and so on;
  the investigating officer who expressed some doubt about the effectiveness of conferences, was most impressed by the process.

In John Braithwaite's terms, this would probably be considered a 'good conference' and in making this evaluation he would apply very different criteria from those used to decide whether a decision of a court was 'good' or 'bad'. It is not the justness or efficiency of the decision which counts, but the participation of the parties and their satisfaction with the process and its outcome.

The second case study involves possession of drugs. This is the way that it was reported:

Background

A 17-year-old male offender was with a group of young people parked in a local park. A police patrol vehicle attended the location in relation to a noise complaint and whilst speaking to the offender, noticed the vehicle was filled with smoke. The offender admitted that the smoke was from a marijuana joint which he had just smoked.

Police intervention

This matter was one that would normally have been placed before the court. One of the concerns of the police officer about using a conference was the question of who was the victim. However, it was decided that a conference was still more appropriate than court.

Caution process

- The offender;
- the offender's parents and two sisters (aged 12 and 15);

- the offender's friend;
- the sergeant as the cautioning officer.

The offender explained the circumstances of the incident. He talked about how he was interested in experimenting with marijuana and how he had managed to purchase some in Melbourne the previous weekend. He said that since the incident, he understood how his actions (and being detected) had impacted upon his family. The offender's father spoke of his son in positive terms but stated that the whole family was having difficulty in coming to accept the fact that 'drugs' were involved. The offender's 15-year-old sister was upset because her brother had been selfish in not considering others.

Outcomes

- The offender apologized to his family for the anguish caused because of his actions;
- he agreed to enter a contract with his parents not to smoke marijuana again;
- both parents said that the incident had brought the family closer together;
- the parents reported later that they felt the conference was a positive and worthwhile experience for the offender and family.

Finally, the author of the case study enigmatically offers as 'issues' the fact that 'this conference challenged the view about victimless crime'. Probably what he means is that, contrary to popular belief, so-called victimless crimes do indeed have victims, namely, the family of the offender. This is interesting, for what this author appears to confuse is the harm caused to the family by the offence, that is, smoking marijuana, and that caused by the fact of its illegality. In this case it was not any direct physical or psychological effects of the smoking that created 'victims', but the construction of smoking marijuana as a crime and the interpretation of the young man's behaviour, not simply as a criminal act, but also as an act which, because it was illegal, demonstrated an indifference to the feelings of members of his family. The threat to family cohesion was, therefore, a product of a law which declared the smoking of marijuana illegal. The meaning or significance of the smoking for the family lay in its illegality. It was this that caused the irritation to the family group, which required remedial or therapeutic measures. Within a system of meaning constructed by law the act was the harm which damaged family relationships. If the family members responded in such a way as to suggest that there was nothing wrong with using marijuana, their condonation would have implicated them in the crime. The family itself would have been regarded as deviant or anti-social and the boy's use of the drug would probably have ended in court. What emerges, therefore, is a conception of good families and bad families, which rests upon the respect of family members for the law. Any deviancy in family attitudes from the meanings generated by the legal system would in this scheme pathologize the family or endow it with a negative value. This would apply to all, not just victimless, crimes. A family which regarded shop-lifting as the fault of shopkeepers for putting temptation in the path of children or drink-induced brawls as youthful high spirits could not expect to be designated as suitable for a family group conference as an alternative to court proceedings. The suitability of the family for the purpose of decision making is, therefore, defined by that family's acceptance of legal constructions of events.

THE PROBLEM OF SOCIAL COMMUNICABILITY

Let us turn now to the other main form of family group conferences which are deployed where children are seen as being in need of some welfare intervention. From a lawyer's perspective what is particularly interesting about the New Zealand experiment is its modification of 'the paramountcy principle' – the idea that the welfare of the child was paramount and it was up to the law (often with the help of psychological experts) to decide where the child's interests lay. The Children, Young Persons and the Families Act, 1989, which set up the family group conferences, removed this paramountcy principle from its central position in decision making about children and introduced in its place the notion of the well-being of children, which is seen as inexorably 'linked to the well-being of their families and family groups' (Webb, 1992, p. 6811).[6] For an observer of autopoietic systems the interest lies not in the abandonment or modification of paramountcy as such, but in the consequential absence of any clear criteria for social judgments. There is no recourse to law or child welfare science which would allow for any decisions emerging from conferences to be judged according either to their lawfulness or to their scientifically-validated benefit to the child. The only ways of knowing whether conference decisions are 'good' or 'bad' are, first, to assess the participation of *whanau* and *hapu* and, second, to find out whether the decision reached had the backing of the family group, and takes into account the child's own wishes. In other words general procedural requirements concerning the convening of the conference and the obtaining of consensus for its decisions take the place of the demands of lawfulness and the scientifically established ways of avoiding harm to children.

It is true that the care of children and their protection from harm emerge as criteria for intervention in Parts II and III of the New Zealand Act, but even here the emphasis is on the primary care and protection role of the family group, on minimizing the necessary interruption to the child's life and on support to the family group to provide care and protection (Swain, 1995, p. 162). As one commentator on the Act reports:

> Removal from the family is only where there is a *serious risk* of harm, it should be as short-term as possible, and where there is not a timely return – with arrangements for protection – to the family group it should be to placement in a *family-like* setting (rather than to an institution, however familial its ambience), such as with relatives or failing that to members of the same *hapu* or *iwi* or ethnic group in the same neighbourhood . . .
>
> (Swain, 1995, p. 162, emphasis added)

An autopoietic theory of closed social systems (see pages 26–29) would have some difficulty in accepting the idea that families or family groups could generate communications at the social level, communications, in other words, which would be recognized by social systems as more than mere noise or perturbation, but as contributing to a stable environment for that system's own communications of certainty and reality. More precisely, in the case of decisions concerning children it is difficult to conceive of a situation in which the function systems of law, economics, politics or science would be able to regard the family or family group as capable of producing authoritative statements about what is good or bad for children, without those statements first being reconstructed according to the coding of one or more of these systems.

In a way this problem has been recognized by the New Zealand legislature, which in 1994 passed the Children, Young Persons and their Families Amendment Act which 'unequivocally reinstated the paramountcy principle' (Swain, 1995, p.161). It 'introduced a new provision that in respect of care and protection matters under the

Act the welfare and interests of the child or young person shall be the first and paramount consideration' (*ibid.*). This leaves child welfare specialists free to determine whether the care arrangements are likely adequately to protect the child and promote his or her welfare. It leaves law able to *know*, through the expert evidence of these specialists, what is legally right and wrong for that child, economics *to know* what are the likelihood of good returns on its investments, and politics to *claim* that vulnerable children, their welfare and interests are being protected by law.

Another way of presenting this same problem of social systems' recognition of what counts as communication is to identify what is not communicable and so must remain for the time being at the general or non-specific level, capable of doing no more than irritate or perturb social systems. This is the same as asking what can be left relatively safely in the realm of noise or uncertainty without being classified as an unacceptable risk and without causing any major disruptions to society. Of course, the existence of any unprocessed noise or lack of certainty is dangerous for social systems, for it may at any time erupt into a major perturbation – the kind of 'moral panic' that criminologists are so fond of describing (see pages 111–112). On the other hand, it is quite impossible for social systems to encode simultaneously every different form or aspect of human behaviour. Selections have to be made and these will be different for different systems at different times. Identifying what is left unselected or unrecognized at any one time by all systems is one possible method of mapping the territory of society's operations, for what is not recognized cannot be 'understood' except in so far as it is recognized as being beyond the realms of understanding. It may well be that the internal operations of *hapu*, *iwi* and *whanu* are seen by politics as existing within this dark realm. What may be important for political accounts is not knowledge about how communities and families operate internally, but merely the existence of these institutions or a belief in their existence. It may be that the fact that these structures can be identified and invoked as potential decision makers is sufficient to imbue the decisions they make with a legitimacy which itself reinforces belief in the existence and importance of these institutions.

However, the limits of tolerance for non-understanding (or noise) clearly do not extend to those situations where the family group or community is asked to respond to behaviour identified by law as 'criminal'. In this case its decisions are assessed according to their pre-ordained meanings for social systems, whether this be in terms of justice, cost-efficiency, or effectiveness in reducing crime. Nor do they extend to those situations where the welfare of the child is seen as paramount, for, as we have seen, what counts as welfare is not left for the determination of the family or group, but has to conform with criteria of acceptability laid down by law and science – the risk of serious or significant harm test.

Where the situation is perceived as one which presents no pressing risk to society or its systems, the tolerance for noise or non-understanding appears to be limitless. The complexity of human relations and the chaotic nature of family (or community) decisions are no bar to legitimacy in such cases. Rather, what appears to matter to political observers is the question whether, by giving the decisions to the family group meeting, 'power' has indeed devolved from 'the state' to 'the citizen', from professionals to the family. Here is a case history from a report on the operation of family group conferences in Winchester, an English cathedral town (Lupton *et al.*, 1995). Here, unlike in New Zealand, the conferences are used only in situations which are *not seen as presenting a significant risk of harm to the child.*

Sophie is a 13-year-old girl living with her mother, step-father, half-sister and brother. She and her immediate family have had no contact with many members of her mother's family, nor with her step-father's family, since she was 5 years old, due to her mother's and step-father's distrust of those family members. Sophie's mother and step-father took her to social services saying that they wanted her put in a children's home because they could no longer control her behaviour. Social services arranged a family group conference (FGC) in the hope that the extended family could find an alternative option to a children's home or foster care.

Sophie's parents were reluctant to participate in the conference, and were adamant that certain family members should not be invited if one was held. Because Sophie wanted some of those family members to attend, however, the coordinator invited all the family members and tried to convince Sophie's parents to come along as well. Not only did Sophie's parents refuse to attend if these other family members attended, the step-father told those family members with whom he was on good terms not to come. He also said that if he and his wife did come, he would post one of his friends at the door to determine who would be allowed into the room. When the FGC was held, the mother and step-father did not attend, nor did any family members they had contacted. Instead, the only family members present were those who had not seen Sophie since she was 5 years old, many of whom did not know each other. At the conference a cousin of Sophie's volunteered to have her live with her, as she had already fostered other children. In addition, the grandfather (Sophie's step-father's father) agreed that Sophie could spend weekends with him.

When the plan was presented to Sophie's parents, they refused to allow it to go through, and informed social services that the grandfather had recently served a prison term related to assault charges. A second conference was held at a later date, with only Sophie, her foster carer and her mother and step-father present. At this FGC a plan was made for Sophie to remain with the carer on a long-term foster care arrangement, with a gradual build up of contact with her parents. While she did remain with the foster carer for some time, her parents made no effort to remain in contact with her and, due to additional behavioural problems, she was eventually moved to another foster home (Lupton *et al.*, 1995, p. 53).

In this case, therefore, the appearance may have been given that 'the family' was empowered. Yet, when the issue of Sophie's future became a matter for the family group conference to decide, 'the family' stopped being 'the family' in the sense of a political symbol and began to be observed as people with different views, beliefs, values, likes, dislikes, histories, interests, desires. The unknowable, the contents of the black box, became known, noise became understandable as interests, desires, likes, dislikes, etc., all of which could be subjected to the scrutiny of researchers, to the analysis of sociologists and psychologists, experts in 'power' and in 'relationships'. As soon as their operations began to be observed using the perspective of social function systems other than politics, the cohesive units of 'family' and 'community', that Braithwaite and others claim to see as providing proof of the enormous value of communitarianism and republicanism in solving social problems, are seen to fragment and disappear.

Atkin, in a commentary on the New Zealand scheme, expresses some of the concerns from these observations when he asks:

how are administrators to know which *hapu* should be consulted when many people belong to more than one *hapu*? What if the

child or young person, or even the birth parents strongly object to bringing the *whanu* or *hapu* into the decision-making process?
(Atkin, 1988–1989, p. 236)

This is not in any way to suggest that all family group conferences are so fraught with difficulties as Sophie's. Indeed, the same report gives accounts of a number of successful conferences where members of the extended family agreed to take some part in looking after a child. The point of these comments is not to dispute the claim that families, family groups or communities may from time to time act in unison. It is rather to argue that, even where this happens, they are not, and cannot be seen as, performing as an autonomous decision makers capable of producing stabilizing and reassuring messages to society and its subsystems. On the contrary, only a re-coding of their operations and their communications in the terms of social function systems is able to provide these comforting messages. As soon as the family group conference is transformed from a symbol of anti-colonialism, anti-statism, anti-legalism, and from an icon for community power and family responsibility – a product of political theorizing – into an instrument for producing decisions about children and young people, it inevitably find its performance observed and evaluated according to what at the time constitute social system constructions of justice, children's welfare, risk, harm, punishment and so on.

CONCLUSION

The observer of systems is not such a deterministic or conservative creature as some readers might have begun to suspect. S/he does not propose that the criteria or values according to which conferences or any other form of decision making are assessed are set down for all times and all places. There is plenty of room for change. Indeed, what is adjudged a just solution, in the interests of children's welfare, harmful to children, risky for children, a suitable punishment, etc. in modern society are seen by the systems observer to be in a constant state of change. S/he is just as capable of seeing these changes and appreciating them as the observer who is ideologically committed to making the world a better place. What the systems observer is most reluctant to accept, however, are the assumptions inherent in the philosophical overlay which Braithwaite and his colleagues bring to their account of family group conferences, the idea that by altering a process from formal to informal, involving one group of people rather than another group of people, or one place rather than another place, you change fundamentally the ways in which society conceptualizes itself. For Braithwaite and others to greet the introduction of these conferences as if it heralded the arrival of a new era of communitarianism or republicanism in which the power of the community, the family or the victim will replace that of the state, the government or the court, seems to be little more than a public relations exercise designed to sell conferences throughout the world. Claims that the shaming and degradation of young offenders leads to more effective crime control than conventional courts and punishment (Braithwaite and Mugford, 1994) also seem to owe more to faith in the quality of the product than to any analysis of the complex relationship between law and other social systems, including the family.

This does not mean to say that the introduction of family group conferences is likely to have no effect whatsoever, but that whatever effects they will have on ways of perceiving crime and children's welfare are largely unpredictable. One could argue that the most likely consequence of the efforts of the communitists and familialists is to open up the black boxes of community and family to the observation of those social systems which are functional for society's self-identity. In the terms of political theorists, it could transport them from the private to the public sphere (Ashenden, 1995). The internal operations of 'family' and 'community' in their conferencing activities then become objects for law, science and politics, with each of these systems constructing family group conferences as part of their environment, to be known, understood and controlled in accordance with their own coding.

Far from changing fundamentally the structure of society, the introduction of conferencing, would, according to these predictions, lead only to its accommodation within existing social function systems, at least in so far as it presented an irritation to these systems. 'Families' and 'communities' might appear as decision makers for youth crime, but only within the conceptual framework of a political and a legal system which has pre-defined crime, justice, power, lawfulness, etc. Similarly, conferences may make decisions for the protection of children, but only within a medico-scientific world which has pre-defined what is and what is not harmful for children. Only in those cases which are perceived as touching upon neither legal nor child protection matters, cases which do not enter the public sphere or which do not create major perturbations for law, politics, science or economics, would one expect families and communities as decision makers to be permitted to operate largely unobserved within their respective black boxes. Even here, however, there is always the risk that science might find them interesting objects for research, which could lead eventually to the involvement of other systems. To some extent the cases from the Wagga Wagga project, changes in the New Zealand law and the restricted use of family group conferences in England bear out these general predictions.

Finally, what of the promise of a better world for children and young people that has attracted so many to the idea of family group conferences? If you accept Braithwaite's measures of progress, his criteria for success, the world will appear to have improved. Other measures, such as the levels of state financial assistance to parents before and after the introduction of conferencing, the severity of penalties between courts and conferences, the long-term success or failure of child placements resulting from conferences, may not give such an optimistic impression. Much depends, therefore, on what you choose as the criteria for progress. In addition, there is the related problem of determining what exactly is good and what is bad for children. How do you decide, if you can no longer rely upon science or a moral consensus to make such pronouncements?

NOTES

1 I am referring here specifically to Australia, Canada, South Africa, the United Kingdom and the USA.
2 For example, David Moore (1992), Stephen Mugford (see Braitwaite and Mugford, 1993) and P. Petit (see Braithwaite and Petit, 1990).
3 This is a matter which causes concern among some feminist writers who see women at a serious disadvantage in negotiations with men, since men usually start from a position of economic and physical superiority. Women, it is argued, may well be bullied or persuaded into agreeing to 'deals' which they would have contested and possibly resisted, had the matter gone to court.
4 Other new forms involve the concept of community. In parts of South Africa, for example, community councils have been set up to deal with minor criminal matters.
5 These case studies were compiled by Terry O'Connell and published in Alder and Wundersitz, 1994, pp. 75–86.
6 See Swain, 1995

Chapter 7

Observing children's rights

PREAMBLE

On 1 June 1992 the 'Children's Summit of South Africa' launched its *Children's Charter*. This document begins as follows:

> Realizing that,
>
> all children are created equal and entitled to basic human rights and freedoms and that all children deserve respect and special care and protection as they grow and
>
> Recognizing that,
>
> within South Africa children have not been treated with respect and dignity, but as a direct result of apartheid have been subject to discrimination and racism that has destroyed communities and has disrupted education and social relationships . . .

Reading through the Articles of the Charter it soon becomes clear that what the Children's Summit is demanding is nothing less than a major programme of political and economic reforms using children's rights as a device to add weight and legitimacy to their demands.[1] The Charter sets out over fifty 'rights' to which it claims all children are entitled. These include:

- the right to participate in the government of the country (art 3(4));
- the right to freedom to practise their own religion, culture or beliefs without fear (art 4);
- the right to be protected from all types of violence including: physical, emotional, sexual, state, political, gang, domestic,

school, township and community, street, racial, self-destructive and all other forms of violence (art 5(1));

- the right to be educated about child abuse and the right to form youth groups to protect them from abuse (art 5(5));
- the right to love and affection from their parents and family (art 5(2));
- the right to clothing, housing and a healthy diet (art 5(3));
- the right to clean water and a clean living environment (art 5(4));
- the right to be protected from harmful and toxic substances, such as cigarettes, drugs, and alcohol . . . (art 7(2));
- the right to free and comprehensive health services (art 7(3));
- the right . . . especially in rural areas . . . to be protected from hard labour including farm, domestic or manual labour or any other type of labour (art 8(2)).

In December 1993 the South African government enacted a new, interim constitution for the country.[2] Section 30 of the Act states:

Every child shall have the right

(a) to a name and nationality as from birth;
(b) to parental care;
(c) not to be subject to neglect or abuse; and
(e) not to be subject to exploitative labour practices nor to be required or permitted to perform work which is hazardous or harmful to his or her education, health or well-being.

I do not intend in this chapter to discuss in detail the feasibility of transforming these rights into reality. What I intend to do, however, is to consider the fairly recent social phenomenon of children's rights formulations – the way in which, particularly since the adoption by the United Nations of the Convention on the Rights of the Child in 1989, manifestos for a better world for children have been constructed in the legal or quasi-legal form of rights. Of particular interest to me is the expectation generated by and among children's rights advocates that the legal system will somehow be able to deliver this utopia, that by transforming what amount to moral precepts into law, the matter becomes simply one of having the will to enforce the law against those who hold out against it, the rights-deniers.

Lawyers, both practitioners and academics, have played an important part in this transformation process. Indeed, it is not hard to understand how the promotion of children's rights has in recent times become such a fertile and productive territory for lawyers. First, it is attractive because it enables lawyers to present the law as an instrument able to remedy injustices, either by outlawing the behaviour that causes suffering or by empowering the victims of this injustice – the oppressed and the exploited. Second, because children are often too young to speak for themselves, adults take it upon themselves to speak for them. Even if some children are old enough to speak their minds as individuals, they are very unlikely to function as a coherent group with distinctive aims and policies designed to promote their interests and those of their fellow children. This, of course, leaves the way open for liberally-minded lawyers who strive to create a more just and less imperfect world to take up the cause of children. Of course, in their efforts to give young people a voice they inevitably project onto them their own discontent with today's social order and their wishes for the future. They interpret the 'bad' treatment of children as revealing the evils which characterize our far-from-perfect society and point the way to improvements in the organization of the social world.

Lawyers' involvement in promoting children's rights, then, is not limited merely to extending access to legal expertise, passing on to the younger generation all the undoubted benefits of legal advice and representation. It goes very much further than that, arriving at a point where it appears to be presenting law as an all-powerful force for good in society, capable of creating a new social order through eliminating or reducing harms to the child. According to the legal message, it is able to achieve this by obliging adults, whether individually or collectively in the form of governments, social institutions and commercial enterprises, to treat children with the dignity and respect due to privileged citizens.

INTRODUCTION: OBSERVING SYSTEMS

Observing law and lawyers

Before discussing further this involvement of law and lawyers in the promotion of children's rights, I should make clear the position that I have taken towards children's rights in this chapter. To begin with, I have deliberately abandoned any notion that a commitment to promote the rights of innocent children is in itself politically innocent, and in taking this position I would refute any claim that children's rights advocates should be treated as if they were on the side of the (little) angels and, therefore, immune from comment in other than reverential tones. Observing children's rights, however, is not necessarily a cynical or negative stance to take. To observe children's rights as a strategic device of combining children with rights as a way of drawing attention to and, hopefully, winning support for a list of demands for political and economic action does not amount to an attack on children or indifference to their welfare. I would, however, defend the view that the promotion of children's rights denotes a political and moral engagement of a particular kind and, as such, must be open to comment. What I have sought to do in this chapter, however, is not to mount a direct attack on children's rights and their promoters, but to analyse from a socio-legal perspective the issue of rights for children and their recent reproduction in legal and quasi-legal forms.

What then is meant here by a socio-legal perspective? Although the term socio-legal has been given several different meanings, my use of the term denotes, in the first place, the detachment of a 'scientific' observer from emotionally-charged political debates and, second, a wish to see law as a social phenomenon existing in modern society, and not to be restricted to lawyers' own definitions of what law is and what it is capable of achieving. In the specific case of children's rights it denotes an absence of commitment either to the brave new world envisaged by the rights advocates or to the medium of rights-as-law as the preferred method for bringing that world into existence. I expect that many lawyers reading this article will find it strange that anyone should want to remain detached from all the pain and suffering that today's children experience in many different parts of the world. Why not join up and fight the good cause – the protection, rescue, liberation and empowerment of children? The problem with commitment is that by definition it starts with the presupposition that one particular course of action is good and that other possibilities, including inaction, are necessarily bad. Choosing to be good in such a situation transforms sociology into a moral crusade or a political struggle. To make such a choice is to abandon any hope of a sociology able to offer an approach to issues which is not simply an amplification or extension of an individual commitment to particular political goals. As an individual I may well want the same kind of world for children to grow up in that the children's rights advocates are promoting. To take a commitment to the sociological enterprise seriously, however, is to put such utopian visions to one side.

Socio-legal observation, therefore, does not seek to take refuge from the complexities, paradoxes and ambivalences that abound on the subject of children and their rights by joining the ranks of child savers and child liberationists. To take this route is in effect to condemn the sociological aspect of the enterprise to the status of a moralizing discourse where only good can come from rights-promoting activities and only bad from those who resist these demands. It is to abandon critical judgment by accepting the simple vision of a world where children are always innocent victims and/or powerless pawns and where certain self-selected adults (usually from the ranks of the liberal professions) have been assigned the heroic task of rescuing them by presenting them with rights with which to defend themselves from the evil perpetrated against them. This is not in any sense to argue that children are well able to defend themselves without help from adults, but rather that the very identification of children as a separate group needing rights to rescue them from the evils of contemporary society involves a series of selections, constructions and distinctions, which sociology has an obligation to recognize. As Ulrich Beck points out:

> The child is the source of the last *remaining, irrevocable, unchangeable primary relationship.* Partners come and go. The child stays. Everything that is desired, but not realizable in the relationship is directed to the child. . . . The excessive affection for children, the 'staging of childhood' which is granted to them – the poor, overloved creatures – and the nasty struggle for the children during and after divorce are some of the symptoms of this. The child becomes the *final alternative to loneliness* that can be built up against the vanishing possibilities of love.
>
> (Beck, 1992, p. 118, emphasis in original)

In short, the socio-legal observer, unlike the lawyer, is unable to take for granted the phenomenon of childhood and the desire to give children rights.[3]

Sociological observation

As I suggested at the start of this book (pages 15-16), the principal task for sociological observers is to create a model of social life which takes account, as far as possible, of the complexities of the social world. It is certainly not an easy task. It involves, for example, including all those political and economic 'realities' which philosophers and jurisprudential scholars, with their eyes on higher, more abstract matters, are so adept at avoiding.[4] How to achieve this and yet remain a detached observer of society, uncommitted to any particular values or scheme for improving society has caused considerable problems for social theorists.

In this chapter I have adopted a theoretical approach which, far from denying subjectivity or concealing it behind a veil of statistical data, rejects the possibility that there can be anything other than subjective values. It is the approach which I described in Chapter 1 and which sees the phenomenal world, the world which we believe to exist, which has meaning for us, as being wholly constructed. Construction occurs at two distinct levels, the psychic and the social, and it is the interaction between them which, at the level of individual consciousness, provides people with the information they need to make sense of the external world and themselves within that world.[5] It allows them to make choices and commit themselves to certain beliefs and values. Of course, we are back again with the problem of commitment, although this time, thanks to recently-developed systems theory, within a theoretical framework which recognizes its limitations as an instrument of analysis. Nevertheless, for the sociological observer to use himself or herself or other individuals as the point of entry into this constructed world is to agree to operate within the limits of that individual's vision of what exists and what is relevant and important.[6]

The solution to this problem may be found in taking 'the social' rather than 'the psychic' or consciousness as the starting point for a theoretical scheme. This offers the idea of a social system which consists of constructions arising out of communications, not at the level of individual interaction, but at that of society.[7] Society, according to this theoretical scheme, consists of communications and nothing but communications.[8] Furthermore, we can separate social communications from communications between individuals by relating the former to the structures that exist in particular historical moments for producing meaning, for making sense of raw phenomena in ways which allow a notion of society to exist and to reproduce itself. In modern society, unlike the hierarchical and stratified organization of former times, communications are principally structured according to functionally differentiated subsystems, such as law, religion, science, politics and economics. Society has evolved in such a way as to vest the communications of certain of these functionally differentiated subsystems with an authority which makes them essential to society's existence. Any decision, for example, which is to carry weight or recognition has to have been reached on the basis of the knowledge and according to the processes of any one of these subsystems.

How then do social systems deal with morals values and principles? Social systems, as I have explained (Chapter 1) are not conscious beings, but are restricted in their knowledge and understanding of their environment by their selectivity, that is, by the choices available to them through their coding. The dilemma, therefore, for the conscious observer, that of wanting to know what is meaningful, true and valid, but at the same time of not wanting to embrace unreservedly any particular moral or political vision, becomes for social systems more or less manageable. Meaning, truth or validity become what is meaningful, true or valid *within the system*, for the system alone. Information from outside the legal system, for example, cannot enter the system as raw data – a bank statement or a psychiatric report on a child have no meaning for law on their own. Instead, they have to be coded by the system – that is, given meaning within the system's programmes. The political system, for instance, selects from its environment those communications which are capable of having meaning within its coding of government/opposition, and these are reconstituted according to the system's programmes relating to the obtaining and retention of power. For economics the coding will be property/no property or profit/loss and the programmes will relate to money. For law the coding is lawful/unlawful or legal/illegal, while its programmes are concerned with the application of the lawful/unlawful distinction to events in its environment and the production of communications based on this distinction. This is the notion of 'operative closure' (Luhmann 1988, 1990 and 1992). It is the system's programmes, therefore, which operate upon the selectively coded information and produce communications for both internal and external consumption. Where social organizations are concerned, these communications are usually in the form of decisions, which become part of the environment for other organizations, available for reconstruction by those organizations, according to their specific coding of the external world. For example, political decisions, when reconstructed in the form of legislation, enter the legal system as law, that is, subject to internal legal forms and processes. The law may interpret statutes in ways which restrict or even negate the intention of the legislators or it may decide to what extent these intentions should be put into effect. Politics, therefore, has no control over law once its decisions have taken on a legal form. All it can do is to make further political decisions to rectify law's misreadings of political communications.

This disassociation of law and politics is not just a constitutional matter concerning the separation or powers. The same interference occurs whenever information from one system crosses the boundary into another system.[9] Political decisions, for example, when reconstituted in economics, do not remain political communications but may become translated, for example, into falls and rises in the prices of shares. The legal system selects what is amenable to legal understanding and arrives at a decision by applying its own internal norms. Religious principles come to be reconstituted within law as legal rights to worship and perform religious rituals (King 1995a and b). Perhaps more importantly for this Chapter on children's rights, legal communications suffer the same fate when they are reconstructed within politics, economics, science, etc. This theoretical scheme, therefore, encourages the observer to concentrate attention on the relationship between the system and its environment and to accept as part of that system's environment communications produced by other systems.

Obviously this process of producing meanings for society through system selections involves on the one side a reduction in complexity, as the system excludes information that it is unable to understand through the application of its coding, and simplifies other information in ways that make it amenable to the operations of the system's programmes. On the other side, however, within the system, the system's struggle to reduce communications from its environment to meaningful proportions has the effect of increasing internal complexity. This in turn generates more and more complex communications for other systems to decipher and so increases their own internal complexity. The processes and procedures, rules and regulations, intricacies and variations in the organization of the legal system are just one example of such internal complexity.[10]

CHILDREN'S RIGHTS AS CRITIQUE

The task of observing sociologically the phenomenon of children's rights should not be confused with that of taking a critical stance towards law and lawyers merely on the ground that law simplifies the complexities of the world. This may well be true, *but then so do all other social systems*. The observer's task, therefore, also requires a watchful approach towards notions of children's rights which rely upon other forms of reductionism than that of law. We need to be careful, for example, of claims by psychologists for universal psychological rights of the child.[11] The fact that images of children and assessments of their psychological needs appear to change often in quite fundamental ways over time, should make the observer cautious about taking seriously any claims that children's needs can be identified in isolation from the particular cultural setting in which children live (Boydon, 1990). The concentration in this chapter on legal solutions to the moral agenda set by children's rights charters is justified by the strength of the children's rights movement among lawyers and the attractiveness of the vision that law is able to convey of establishing a new order for children through the medium of legal and quasi-legal instruments (Freeman, 1995).

Just as one should be watchful of the problem-solving claims of professional groups, be they lawyers or psychologists, one should also be suspicious of simple accounts of children and their rights which rely upon romantic accounts of children and childhood. One such account sees children as Rousseauesque creatures, with their intuitions intact, uncorrupted by knowledge of the adult world. Today Wordsworth's *Preludes*, Blake's *Songs of Innocence and of Experience* and Rousseau's *Emile* are hardly likely to be widely read and even less likely to be studied as serious statements about a-world-we-have-lost.[12] Childhood and children tend to be perceived in less idealized ways. Nevertheless, the notion of the child as 'noble savage' still persists among some educationalists, psychoanalysts and, indeed, among some advocates of autonomy rights for children. If, as these child rights advocates propose, children can be relied upon to know 'intuitively' what is best for them,[13] then there is no need for children's rights to be anything other than the expression of the needs and desires that can be found within children themselves. The role of the children's rights advocate would be to identify these needs and desires by listening to 'the inner child' (e.g. Kroll, 1994, 1995) and then to set about changing the child's world in order that those needs and desires might as far as possible be met. This leaves the committed children's rights advocate the relatively easy task of identifying the obstacles that exist to this childhood utopia and how they might be overcome.

Seeing children and their rights in this way may have a seductive charm for critics of the evils of modern society. Its problem is, however, that it completely denies complexities rather than confronts them. Once one departs from the radicalism of Rousseau and moves towards the kind of approach which advocates that the wishes of children should generally be tempered by an adult evaluation as to whether those wishes are 'reasonable' and are really likely to promote the best interests of the child, it is no longer possible to avoid complexities. Any evaluation of the reasonableness of children's wishes leads back inevitably to complexity and in particular to the necessity of adults using moral, political, scientific, or legal norms[14] to reduce this complexity to manageable proportions and so to allow them to make decisions as to what is good and bad for children. And this, of course, does require some prior knowledge of society.

As I suggested at the start of this chapter, in order to situate the children's rights movement as existing within a society of communications produced by closed social systems, we need first to distance ourselves from the idea that rights for children has been created through the hard work of well-intentioned people committed to making the world a better place for the young. Instead, the task that I am proposing is to examine the phenomenon of children's rights as the unlikely product of co-evolving social systems. This would start with the recognition that the concepts of 'children' and 'rights' are able to exist in combination with one another only where both have achieved a level of significance to allow them to operate in a generalized way across the semantic boundaries of several different social systems. This generalized existence signals the acceptance, first, of the distinction between child and adult as denoting that the young are not just little or embryonic adults, or merely members of a family, but have achieved the status of a social group distinguished from adults through the imposition of an arbitrary age barrier (now generally 18 years).[15] It is a distinction which law, politics, religion, the psychological sciences and economics have all played a part in creating. All of these subsystems find themselves obliged to take their creation seriously, for failing to do so is likely to threaten the fragile interdependence which holds them, and thus society, together. One can imagine the disruption that would occur if, tomorrow, 12-year-olds were permitted to leave school, and enter full-time employment, or if they were granted the right to vote in elections, to marry, to fight wars, regularly to sue adults (including their own parents), or to invest in the stock market. The retention of the distinction between adult and child, therefore, is not simply a legal construction, but has significance for the programmes of all those systems which modern society has designated as sites of authority.

When we examine closely the notion of rights in the light of this child/adult distinction we find that it contains within itself a central paradox. This paradox is that giving children rights has the effect of drawing attention to the fact that children cannot expect to have equal rights to adults. It serves to reinforce the adult/child distinction, while at the same defining children not only as vulnerable, but also as privileged citizens. It is the very inequality and the continuation of this inequality between children and adults which gives children, so to speak, a right to rights. Children have rights because they do not have, and cannot be expected to have, *full citizen's rights*.

Of course, it is the vulnerability of children to adult exploitation, corruption, violence and oppression, which most child-rights advocates would argue makes the recognition of these rights so essential in the modern world. It is this child-protective aspect that receives most attention in children's rights legal formulations. The image of the suffering child comes to symbolize all the injustices of the world, while giving rights to children seems to offer a way of protecting children against all those injustices. It is not by chance that the children's rights movement has put so much faith in the transformation both nationally and internationally of children's rights into *legally constituted rights*. Science, medicine and education may claim to be able to identify the positive factors that make for happy and fulfilled children, and the negative factors which prevent and inhibit the development of the healthy child. But what authority do these subsystems possess to enable them to oblige adults to behave in ways which promote children's well-being? In the absence of any authority external to society, such as that provided by a universal belief in an obligation to obey God's commandments, and given the extreme difficulties in modern society of reformulating personal morality at the level of social communications,[16] only law of all the social subsystems claims for itself the capacity to rectify injustices, and to provide those normative values which avoid the necessity for people to learn from experience (Luhmann, 1986, 1989a; Teubner, 1992). Within law, precepts about what is good and what is bad for children may be given the authority of the legal system's lawful/unlawful coding. Once formulated as law, therefore, children's rights may be used to identify conduct by adults, whether individually or collectively in the form of governments or social institutions, which causes harm to children, and to condemn such conduct as illegal and its perpetrators as law-breakers.

Seen in this light, it is not perhaps surprising that the *United Nations Convention on the Rights of the Child*, and all the other constitutional instruments which seek to set down rights for children, tend to generate legal communications that go far beyond the scope of what is recognizable as law. Indeed, even to see them as law is something of a misreading. They are formulated as law, because and only because there is no other mode (or code) for modern society to make generally available its fears and hopes for children and their future and, at the same time, to hold out the possibility of allaying those fears and realizing those hopes. The romantic Christian idea that children who die in childhood can expect to play together for eternity in a heavenly paradise no longer has any credence. Similarly, the belief that people's lives are foreordained according to some grand scheme denies (or at least limits) any possibility of the forging of a causal connection between present child and future adult. In modern society this belief has been replaced by a scientific (and now common-sense) equivalence between childhood well-being and adult well-being, which tells us that the future destiny of our children lies in   present decisions.[17] Accordingly, happy and fulfilled children would appear to make for happy and fulfilled adults. This message concerning the relationship between the child and the adult, the present and the future, may well be common to all the subsystems of modern society. Of these, however, only law has the capacity to reconstitute this relationship in the form of rights and obligations. Adults can *through law* be required to make sacrifices in order to make children and the future happy and secure. They may even *through law* be made to suffer penalties if they fail to meet their obligations.

The reason for this faith in the power of law may stem more from a disillusionment and a lack of faith in other systems, such as politics, economics, science and religion, to protect children and their future well-being than from any widespread popularity of law or lawyers. Contemporary politics in both democratic and autocratic countries, both nationally and internationally, provides little evidence of its ability to treat children as a distinctive group, separate from adults and families, deserving preferential treatment. Indeed, many would claim that the greatest harm recently to be inflicted on children comes from the domestic policies of political parties or the foreign policies of national governments.[18] Economics presents children as assets or liabilities, consumers and potential producers of wealth. The notion of pupils and students as human capital, for example, underpins much of the economics of education.[19] Restricted as it is to seeing the world in these cost-benefit terms, it can hardly be expected to adopt the welfare of all children as one of these benefits. Scientific discoveries may reveal the risks that abound in childhood, but science and its discoveries are also responsible for creating some of those risks. Moreover, all that science is able to do is to discover scientific truth; it is unable to make the decisions about what is good or bad, right or wrong for children. Religion may at one time have protected children and promoted their welfare, but now religious practices may be seen as harming children and restricting their freedoms rather than protecting them, and promoting their autonomy.[20]

It is probable, therefore, that the present popularity of internationalism and constitutionalism in law expresses not only a general desire for a binding global and national order coupled with guarantees for individuals and minority groups, but also a recognition that law is all that is now available to modern society for the task of creating such moral communities. The recent surge of treaties, conventions, charters and constitutions may be seen almost as a symbolic denial that society has gone beyond the point at which it is possible to appeal to a moral consensus. Within law, and only within law, is the impression of a consensus still possible.

Furthermore, what may give law a special popularity among rights enthusiasts is the fact that, unlike other systems, such as politics, economics and science, it appears capable of regulating its own affairs. Law extends its reach inwards to law itself, with international conventions and state constitutions, etc. being formulated as meta laws, laws that have the capacity to regulate not only people and institutions, but also other laws. Seen in this light, the children's rights formulations, as they appear in national and international conventions and constitutions, give the misleading impression of offering a universal (or national) moral code for the treatment of children. Necessarily, this involves a constructive misreading of law's capabilities. Attributing to law in modern society a greater authority than any other of society's function systems to determine what is right and wrong is to misread legality as denoting simultaneously both what is morally acceptable and what is, according to current scientific knowledge, healthy for children. Yet in practice all that law can do is to decide what is right and wrong *in law*, that is *what is lawful and what is unlawful, what is legal and what is illegal.* This may or may not correspond to what people believe to be moral and immoral. There is certainly no guarantee that it will do so. Moreover, the more ambitious international and constitutional law becomes and the more culturally diverse the populations of nation states, the less likely it is that law will represent universal or national moral standards.

One other effect of this misreading is the confusion between children's legal rights and children's absolute welfare, making it appear as if there can always be definitive determinations as to what is good for the child, and that promoting children's rights as legal requirements will necessarily result in improvements in child welfare. Conversely, any denial of legal rights for children is likely to be misinterpreted as necessarily bad for children and the future of society. In these circumstances to speak out against the legal and quasi-legal formulations of children's rights to be found in conventions, constitutions, charters, etc. becomes the modern-day equivalent of nailing a list of protestations to the doors of a cathedral. It risks situating the protester outside the existing legal, moral and scientific orders.

THE CLOSED SYSTEM OF CHILDREN'S LEGAL RIGHTS

A political scientist observing the evolution of the campaign for children's rights might well question the basic presuppositions upon which much of rights communications appear to be based. These seem to assume the existence of a nation state or world community operating as a cohesive entity or, alternatively, they assume that it is possible to impose such cohesion through the medium of law. Only by accepting one or other of these assumptions, the political scientist might well argue, is it possible to ignore the many divergent and often conflicting interest groups, cultural, religious and customary divisions that exist in the modern world, to say nothing of the huge gap in life-styles between the richer and the poorer nations and between the rich and the poor within the same national boundaries. If the hope of those responsible for drafting international conventions and state constitutions and charters on children's rights is that these instruments will operate as a rallying cry for all the peoples of the world (or nation) to put aside their differences and join together in creating a better future for children, it is likely to run headlong into the realities of national and global politics as well as those of state and international economic institutions. Similarly, the idea that governments or religious or cultural groups which ignore or contest children's rights will somehow be coerced or shamed into conforming with all the Articles of the Convention is likely to appear unduly optimistic.

Yet simply to dismiss the children's rights endeavour as naïve or misguided seems both cynical and inadequate as a response to a worldwide movement which has caught the imagination of many people, including very many lawyers. If the project was indeed doomed to failure from the start, how could it attract so much support and enthusiasm? It is precisely here that closed systems theory is able to offer an explanation. A brief glance at the historical accounts of the gestation of the *United Nations Convention on the Rights of the Child*, the inspiration for much of today's children's rights endeavours, demonstrates how what are now accepted as children's rights in international law resulted in fact from long and protracted negotiations and debates between representatives of nation states and of non-governmental organizations (NGOs) claiming knowledge and expertise on children and their welfare (Cohen, 1990; Alston *et al.*, 1992; Alston, 1994 and King 1994).

The enormous achievement of all those engaged in producing the Convention cannot be overestimated. However, once the decision had been taken to formulate children's rights as international law, the objective became not that of finding solutions to highly complex problems, often involving an enormous range of interrelated factors. Instead, what had to be accomplished was the creation of law in the form of a piece of international legislation, namely the Convention. The task undertaken by the United Nations Working Group became one of translating general principles into a formula that would be acceptable to all the governmental delegations – one, in other words, of law making (Cohen, 1990). The expectation was that, once the Convention had been adopted by the United Nations Organization and ratified by most of the countries of the world, there would be a strong incentive for individual governments and the world community to find solutions to specific problems concerning children.

Unfortunately, this hope could never be fully realized, for reasons that I have already discussed. It was based on a misreading of law's capacities, an unquestioning acceptance of law's self-generated identity as having supreme authority over all society's activities. Moreover, the drafters of the Convention were further misled by the communications of international law into thinking that those nation states which ratified the Convention were capable of controlling all child-harming activities within their territories, and that the creation of a child-friendly world order was thus just a matter of securing the agreement of these nations to obey international law. Nation states, within the political rather than the legal system, however, consist only of governments. Governments not only represent, but they also act in the name of, the nation state while they are in office. Since power is limited in time to their period in office, governments are continually engaged in the task of trying to hold on to power, to retain office – a task which ends only when they cease to be a government.[21] This is the case whether the government is oligarchical or democratic. Only the methods of gaining and retaining power are different, the first depending on the active suppression of all opposition and the second by convincing the electorate that it is better equipped than the opposition to deal with the pressing problems that are creating anxiety for voters.[22]

In much the same way that the belief – held by the multi-national children's rights advocates who drafted the Convention – that regulation of nations' behaviour towards their children was achievable through international law, was a misreading of *law's construction of reality* as absolute reality, so the Children's Summit of South Africa, which adopted the *Children's Charter of South Africa*, misread the country's political and economic systems as consisting of people and nothing else. Since people's behaviour is seen by law as capable of being regulated and controlled by law, so, according to this logic, could these systems. In this way making constitutional-like declarations of children's rights would not only hold up to the government a set of ideals which could be achieved through the regulation and control of people, it would also act as a measure against which the South African government and the country's provincial governments' performance in promoting children's welfare could be assessed. Unfortunately for such regulatory ambitions, social systems in modern society do not consist just of people and cannot be regulated by law as if they did. A theoretical strategy which distinguishes people from systems and interpersonal communications from communications at the level of social systems, does, I suggest, help to avoid this kind of misreading and enable the observer to confront complexities to which ideologically-bound endeavours are blind.

As Gunther Teubner (1993, p. 74) has pointed out, the autopoietic notion of the closed system has far-reaching consequences for regulation through law. What it means is that one can no longer rely upon the input–output model which has characterized much of the thinking about law's role in society. The direct intervention which this model proposes is no longer a possibility, since the legal (and any other) system does not have access to the environment (or reality) but only to 'its own internal construction of that environment'. Therefore, 'we must abandon notions of linear causation, where legal norms bring about social change directly' (*ibid.*).

All that appears possible for law is self-regulation, i.e. controlling the environment that law has itself constructed. This is in itself unlikely to affect the operations of other systems, and may even give rise to unintended consequences, when legal communications are reconstructed within those systems. Constitutional declarations outlawing the employment of children, for example, are likely to be interpreted within the economic system in terms of cost–benefits. The illegality of employing children is likely to be constructed by economics as a risk – that of prosecution and financial sanctions – to be set against the obvious economic benefits of continuing to employ children. If some industries important for the country's exports depend for their profitability upon child labour, the government is also likely to reconstruct the law in economic terms when it decides whether or not to enforce the law. Since, governments today are likely to be held responsible for the country's economic performance in world markets, political considerations may well be structurally linked to economic policies concerning the enforcement of the law.

The other possibility which Teubner discusses is regulation through indirect intervention. This is similar to Luhmann's notion that to plan 'action contexts' (i.e. systems) may meet with more success than to plan only actions because:

> Such systems can be controlled by planning, or possibly even created. However, the planner cannot replace action itself; he can only make decision-making premises for others' action and at the most have some foresight regarding the constellation of other decision-making premises to which his own could be adapted. This foresight may be helped by the fact that he imagines the action to be a system, and plans and researches it as a system.
>
> (Luhmann, 1985, p. 271)

Children's rights charters, conventions and constitutional clauses generally take the form of demands and exhortations for actions directed against harms to children or restrictions on their freedoms.

They attempt to impose on government(s) the responsibility for ensuring that these actions are in fact enacted, although there is usually no clear indication as to what will happen to governments if they fail in this responsibility and children continue to be harmed.[23] Autopoietic theory would predict that, given the normatively closed nature of social systems and the impossibility of direct input–output relations, the effective regulation of harmful behaviour to children through this method is unlikely to succeed, for it relies upon a vision of society which exists and continues to be reproduced within (and only within) those closed systems which have no way of 'seeing' or 'understanding' the complexities of inter-system regulation in modern society. In the next section of this chapter, I shall be looking at those ways in which the Luhmann/Teubner notions of system planning and regulation may be applied to the treatment of children. In order to make this conceptual leap, however, one needs to abandon the rights discourse and to concentrate instead on those harms which are most likely to blight the lives of children, and then ask how it might be possible, through indirect intervention or 'system planning' or system creation, to reduce them.

HARMS TO CHILDREN

If we search globally for the causes of the most widespread and most severe suffering to children, we find not deliberate acts by adults to cause children harm, but rather such general calamities as war, disease, poverty, natural disasters and family breakdown. Even if we restrict our search to the harmful effects of government decisions, we hardly ever find that there was any deliberate intention to damage children. Within the party politics of democratic systems any government which openly treated children with callousness or indifference would soon lose the support of the electorate. Even dictators need to give the impression that the welfare of the nation's children is close to their hearts. Where government policies clearly harm children, it is often because the children harmed are not considered *as children*, but as members of or closely connected to a group which a government seeks to defeat or control, such as 'the enemy', 'illegal immigrants' or 'criminals'. The social and economic disadvantages that many children suffer could, for example, be avoided if prison sentences were excluded for all offenders who were participating in their children's upbringing at the time of their trial, but no one, not even the most enthusiastic children's rights advocate, would seriously suggest that this should be government policy. In addition, policies which benefit some children may harm others. The health of children who live on traffic-polluted streets is likely to improve if private cars were banned, but the children who travel regularly in these cars would be likely to have their lives restricted. Harms to children may arise also from a government's determination to keep to a particular ideological agenda, which it believes will restore the fortunes of the nation and by doing so convince the electorate of its integrity. This does not mean that there are never any ways of avoiding or alleviating the harm, but rather that simple legal solutions, such as declaring laws, conduct or decisions to be unlawful because they contravene children's rights, are unlikely to make much impact on harmful conduct towards children, even in those parts of the world where war, famine and disease are not problems.

Serious harm to children may result from economic activities which individual governments, faced with the task of creating wealth through success in world markets, are reluctant to control for fear that it would reduce the nation's competitiveness. This may not just be a cynical disregard for humanitarian values, but may be based on a belief that everyone in the country, including children, will benefit if the economy is thriving. Harms to children may also be caused by mismanagement or inefficient management of the economy, resulting in job losses, long-term unemployment and the probability of family disruption and dislocation. To eliminate such harms will often require major programmes of reform resulting in social upheavals which themselves could have unintended adverse consequences for children.

Two further general points emerge from this examination of serious harms to children. In the first place, only in those countries divided by internal strife are you likely to find governments that deliberately target certain groups, which may include children, for repressive and harmful state action. Most other governments firmly believe themselves to be promoting political programmes which benefit the children living within their territories. The second point is that the most general and far-reaching improvements in children's lives are likely to come about only as the result of a general amelioration in living conditions, the control of disease, the redistribution of wealth, high levels of employment, educational provision, etc. These improvements involve complex forces, often today on a global scale, over which both individuals and individual governments can expect to have only limited control.

SYSTEM PLANNING

The clear message is not that governments can never be obliged or
persuaded to reduce any of the harms inflicted on children within
their territories, but rather that the scope for change through the
imposition of direct legal intervention is extremely limited. As might
be expected from autopoietic theory, children's rights are likely to be
most successful where they operate within the boundaries of the system and can be incorporated in that system's programmes. Within
law the imposition of procedural rights and obligations is an internal legal process. Many of the judgments of the European Court
and recommendations of the European Commission for Human
Rights in favour of extending children's rights have involved increasing the procedural protections, the due process rights of children –
ensuring that there is a judicial hearing before parents are prevented
from demanding the return of their children voluntarily in care,[24] or
before they are refused access to their children by social services,[25]
and that children who have been in care should have access to their
case records. Clearly, for law these rights are important in that they
help to avoid procedural injustices. Whether they reduce the chances
that ultimately the decisions taken by courts and administrative
bodies will cause harm to children is much less clear. Where decisions of the Court and Commission go beyond procedural justice
and require changes in the substantive treatment of children, these
are often controversial, raising doubts among many people as to
whether these changes are necessarily beneficial to children.[26]

From the perspective of Luhmann's notion of systems planning
and Teubner's indirect intervention, what is interesting about the
few successes that have been achieved for children's rights promotion through the procedures of the European Human Rights
Convention is that they involved the 'structural coupling'[27] of law
and politics. The terms of the Convention ensure that the Court's
decision or the settlement between the parties results in an 'irritation' for governments, imposing a political and legal obligation on
the government found to have committed a human rights violation
to change its laws in order to avoid future violations. This obligation provides for the co-evolution of legal and political programmes
around the decisions of the European Human Rights Court and
Commission. Responsibility for any unpopular changes in domestic
legislation and administrative practice can thus be passed from the
national government to the Commission or Court. Where no such

structural couplings exist, as in the case of the *United Nations Convention on the Rights of the Child*, this displacement of political responsibility is not possible. This was brought home recently when the United Nations Committee on the Rights of the Child condemned the United Kingdom government's record in respecting and promoting the articles of the UN Convention. As autopoietic theory predicts, the legal communications of the Convention become reconstructed within other systems *in terms that make sense to those systems*. It was not surprising then to find the British government responding in legal formalist terms to the United Nations requirement for reporting on the progress within its territory of children's rights[28] or to hear politicians from the ruling Conservative Party accuse the United Nations of trying to impose alien values upon the British people.[29] In the absence of any structural coupling between law and politics, therefore, complaints from legal or quasi-legal international organizations about violations of children's rights become reconstructed not as legal duties but as threats to national government and seen as unjustified and ill-informed criticism that the government is unable or unwilling to fulfil its international or constitutional obligations. The obvious political response of governments is to defend themselves against these charges by denying them, thus undermining the authority of their accusers. Only where absolutely necessary do they respond by complying with their international obligations. But even here the changes that they introduce are likely to take the form of cosmetic reforms in the law, which are unlikely to affect the governments' political objectives. What they are least likely to do is to take substantive measures to improve children's lives (even if this were possible), where these would conflict with their political programmes or compromise the ideological stance that won them the confidence of the electorate or those parts of the electorate on which they rely for their support.

In the same way, where no structures exist coupling law with economics in a way that produces the desired outcomes through manipulation of costs and benefits, attempts to impose children's rights directly upon economic institutions are likely to lead to a reconstruction of legal regulations in ways which minimize their effects upon the economic order. To put it crudely, just as support for children's rights is not likely to win votes for politicians, it is unlikely to make money for bankers, stockbrokers or international corporations. This is not to say that nothing that financial institutions do is ever likely to be of benefit to some children, but rather that these benefits will be the normal consequences of existing economic programmes and not the result of attempts through the law to impose children's rights obligations upon these institutions.[30]

Changes within the economic system are much more likely to result from economic incentives and disincentives than from appeals based on morality or child protection. When the Shell oil company recently changed its decision not to sink the redundant Brent Spar oil platform in the North Sea, in spite of the legality and political acceptability of this manoeuvre, the incentive for the change of policy came largely from a widespread boycott by individual consumers of Shell products. A similar attempt to regulate conduct harmful to children through a similar consumer boycott of carpets produced through child labour, however, has proved unsuccessful. While this kind of direct economic action may occasionally be effective, therefore, its effects tend at best to be haphazard and unpredictable. Where the goods are available internationally, the boycott has to be global in order to work.[31] Moreover, consumers probably need to be convinced that alternative products are available (as was the case in the Shell boycott), so that their own economic interests are not likely to suffer.

One could envisage the possibility of effective regulation through structural coupling or system planning of very specific economic conduct which damages children's lives. Remaining with our example of child labour in carpet manufacturing, it would theoretically be possible for governments to introduce direct economic incentives by, for example, subsidizing carpet manufacturers who did not employ children, or paying families for sending their children to school. For this to happen, however, there would have to be some political motive for governments to act in this way. Similarly, the law could be coupled with the system of market manufacturing. All hand-made carpet manufacturers, distributors and retailers could enter into a binding legal agreement not to employ people under a certain age and to set up an enforcement agency to ensure that the agreement was respected. Alternatively, a specific prohibition on the employment of children in this industry and on the sale of carpets manufactured using child labour could be introduced as international law and enforced through the seizure of stocks and the imposition of financial penalties for any contravention, much like the existing prohibition on the production and sale of goods made from ivory. In both cases there would need to be sufficient financial incentives or disincentives for the law to operate effectively and these costs and benefits would need to take into account the operation of the complex system of carpet manufacture and distribution and not assume that passing laws forbidding child labour would achieve their objective.

This may be a far cry from the conceptualizations of problems that characterize the communications of rights activists. Indeed, where attempts have been made to forge structural couplings between law, economics and politics around human rights issues, they have so far failed. An example is the project of making foreign aid to developing nations dependent upon their human rights record.[32] While such strategies may be legally sound in their punishment of the transgressor, they are politically and economically risky. Not only are they likely to rebound on donor nations where those nations have investments and citizens present in the donee country, but they are also likely to harm the very people who would benefit from the continuation of aid and be harmed by its withdrawal. In the case of the infringement of children's rights, the harm to children caused by the withholding of economic aid will probably be more acute than that created by the original rights transgression.

THE LIMITS OF CHILDREN'S RIGHTS AS REGULATION

What conclusion may we now draw from the application of the theory of closed systems to the problems we have identified? For a start the effect of formulating general moral principles on the treatment of children, as international or national constitutional law, is neither as simple nor as beneficial to children as children's rights activists would want us to believe. To commit oneself to a belief in children's rights as law is to accept law's version of a world where the operations of social institutions may be regulated as if they were nothing other than individuals or collections of individuals. It is blind to the internal operations of social communication systems, the inner workings of the black box, or is unable to see them as autopoietic entities operating independently of the people who work in them. Hence, the decisions of political, economic or scientific systems become reconstituted in ways that make them appear amenable to regulation through direct application of law's lawful/unlawful coding. Not only does this serve to reduce the complexities of these systems to terms that legal programmes can 'understand', but it also creates expectations that children's lives, and not just the legal formulations of children's rights, can be improved by these lawful/unlawful decisions. It leads, for example, to the expectation that the inquiries of constitutional courts and the United Nations Committee on the Rights of the Child are actually capable of identifying what is bad for children and, through their decisions or dialogues with national governments, of putting an end to the evil. All that these organizations are able to achieve with any consistency, however, are improvements in and developments of the law concerning children's rights. They are able to operate only upon the second order, legal reconstructions of harms to children and not upon the harms themselves. What effects (if any) these new, improved legal communications are likely to have on children's lives, therefore, are unpredictable and by no means necessarily beneficial to children in every case.

Does this mean that the only path open to us is to throw up our arms in despair and lament the brutality and callousness of a society which turns its back on and even promotes the suffering of innocent children? Certainly not. It does suggest, however, the need for ways of conceptualizing complex social issues, different from those that are offered by human rights and their legal enforcement. The attempts by legal rights lawyers to deal with such difficult issues as pluralism, multi-culturalism and relativism (Alston, 1994; Freeman, 1995) cry out for a more nuanced analysis than that available from law's programmes. Taking, as we have done, the starting point of harm to children, it is then possible, using a closed system approach, to examine how each of those systems, which are treated by society as authoritative, understands and gives meaning to communications from other systems concerning 'harm to children'. 'Systems planning' starts from the premise of observing events in the world as the product of the interrelationships between different autopoietic systems of communication. Once the researcher's task has been modified from that of searching for causes and effects to that of identifying systems and their operations, there is a possibility that the complexity of society and the limitations of direct intervention will be acknowledged. As Niklas Luhmann wrote in an unusually optimistic vein:

> Systems, generally, may control selected facts or events in their own environment related to their own inputs and outputs. They cannot control interdependencies in their environment. The more we rely on systems for improbable performances, the more we shall produce new and surprising problems, which will stimulate

the growth of new systems which will again interpret interdependencies, create new problems, require new systems.

(Luhmann, 1982, p. 134)

The problem then changes its shape. No longer is it a matter of devising legal codes and insisting that other systems are under a legal or moral obligation to obey them. Nor is it one of finding effective methods of enforcing these codes and condemning nation states, their bureaucracies or economic institutions for failing to take children's rights seriously. As long as conceptualizations of harm to children remain in the form of outrages against children's legal rights and the condemnation of these outrages by courts or international bodies, it is not possible for the internal programmes of these institutions to do anything other than misread in ways that make sense to them. If they take them seriously, it will only be in a way that has meaning for the internal communications of closed systems. Put rather more positively, the very most that children's rights activists have the right to expect is for their communications to discourage the most blatantly child-harming operations of market and political forces by attributing a negative value to these operations within the system's programmes, such as loss-making, power-losing, etc. Even here the chances of success are small and, of course, even smaller where the motivation for child-harming activities is the enlargement of territories or the destruction of an internal or external enemy.

NOTES

1   This device was previously employed in relation to South African children in article 10 of the ANC draft Bill of Rights, which states:

> All children shall have the right to a name, to health, to security and to equal treatment . . . the state shall to the maximum of its available resources seek to progressively fulfil the realization of children's rights, that no child shall suffer discrimination or enjoy privileges on the ground of race, colour, gender, language, creed, legitimacy or status of his or her parents, and that in all proceedings concerning children, the primary consideration shall be the best interests of the child . . .

2   Constitution of the Republic of South Africa, Act 200 of 1993. The Act came into operation on 27 April 1994.
3   In the hands of some socio-legal researchers sociology may appear as nothing more than knowledge about how to carry out social research into legal issues. This has proved enormously advantageous to these

researchers who are able to claim that their results possess an objectivity which makes them independent of any personal attitudes or ideological commitments. To make such claims, however, which rest on the reconstitution of sociology as nothing more than research techniques, is to make a virtue out of ignorance. Socio-legal research of this kind becomes a way of not knowing operating rather like the Freudian defence mechanism of denial. What science does not know or recognize cannot affect the (internal) validity of science. See also Jenks, 1996.

4 I am reluctant to name names here, but a glance at some of the essays in Alston, Parker and Seymour (1992) should give some indication of the approach to which I am referring.

5 See, generally, Mead (1934) and Berger and Luckmann (1966).

6 See, generally, Luhmann, 1988.

7 For a full account of the theory see Chapter 1 and, for example, Luhmann, 1977; Luhmann, 1986; King, 1993 and King and Schütz, 1994.

8 Communications consist of three elements: information, utterance and understanding. They of course include decisions as these are the communications of organizations.

9 See Chapter 1.

10 The complexity of the rules of evidence, by which external events become transformed into legal facts, is an example of this process.

11 In the late 1970s the Association of Schools Psychologists decided to work together with the United Nations to produce a Declaration of the Psychological Rights of the Child. This declaration was published following its adoption by the Third Colloquium of School Psychologists on 12 July 1979. The world is still awaiting its implementation (see Catterall, 1980; King, 1982). The recommendation of general suspicion towards claims of universal psychological needs for children extends to claims by lawyers and politicians, who believe that law and politics are able to create the conditions for satisfying children's psychological needs.

12 For a general account of the child as the noble savage, see Fairchild (1928). See also Jenks 1996.

13 Some evolutionary theorists may have taken to wearing Rousseau's mantle in their attribution of survival strategies to children. Refusal to eat green vegetables is, for example, explained as a defence against the poisonous shrubs which grew in the forests of our forefathers' time.

14 The process of learning, not learning from first-hand experience, but from the norms communicated by systems.

15 The fact that 18 years is stated in the *United Nations Convention on the Rights of the Child* as denoting the boundary between childhood and adulthood does not make it any less arbitrary.

16 See Luhmann (1993) and Chapters 1 and 2 of this book.

17 For example, all accounts of 'child abuse survivors' make this explicit connection between childhood abuse and adult suffering. Moreover the psychological literature on sexual and emotional abuse places much emphasis on the long-term effects of such abuse.

18 Even the United Nations has been blamed for harming Iraqi children through its sanctions (Y. Bonnet *Le Monde*, August 1995, translated in *The Guardian*, 9 August 1995).

19 I am grateful to Jean Floud for this example.

20 See the debates concerning female circumcision and also the dissenting opinion of Douglas in *Wisconsin* v. *Yoder* (1972) 406 US 205.

21 See Luhmann (1990) Chapter 5 and also pages 48–52 for a discussion of the autopoietical nature of political systems.

22 This may involve the government successfully defining for the electorate what those problems are in ways that make it appear that it, and only it, has the ability to provide effective solutions.

23 *The European Convention on Human Rights* is an exception to this rule, although, as we shall see, sanctions are likely to extend only to procedural failures rather than to more general failures of protecting children from harm.

24 *R* v. *United Kingdom* (1983), Application No. 10496/83, European Commission of Human Rights.

25 *R* v. *United Kingdom* (1988) FLR 445. See also *W* v. *United Kingdom* (1983), Application No. 9749/82, European Commission of Human Rights.

26 See, for example, the report of the Commission in *Kjeldsen, Madsen and Pedersen* v. *Denmark* (1975), Application Nos. 5095/71, 5920/72 and 5926/72, in which the Commission supported the argument of parents that their children should not be obliged to attend compulsory sex education classes.

27 This involves the co-evolution of system and environment or, more specifically, system and system around certain issues, events or generalized concepts such as rights, agreements, etc:

> A system is structurally coupled to its environment when it uses events in the environment as perturbations in order to build up its own structure. Where a system has internally available the distinction between self-reference and hetero-reference, it may via structural coupling make itself dependent upon its environment by using external events as conditions for its own operations, as irritants or even as opportunities.
>
> (Luhmann, 1989b, p. 8)

> without structural coupling there would be no perturbation and the system would lack any chance to learn and transform its structures.
>
> (Luhmann, 1992, p. 1432)

28 The *Initial Report by the Government of the United Kingdom to the UN Committee on the Rights of the Child* contained several examples of formalistic replies to questions concerning the implementation of children's rights in the UK. For example, in response to Article 37a of the Convention, which sets out the right of children not to be subject to torture or other cruel, inhuman or degrading treatment or punishment, the UK Government replied that in the United Kingdom

'courts have no power to order any form of cruel or degrading treatment or punishment to young offenders'.

29 The Conservative Member of Parliament, and Parliamentary
Representative for the Police Federation, Ivan Lawrence, argued in a
BBC television discussion of the UK Government's children's rights
record that reasonable corporal punishment in private schools should
be allowed to continue without interference from international bodies,
because it represented parental choice as to the way they wished their
children to be educated and disciplined and that there was no evidence
that this traditional way of treating children caused them any harm.

30 If one takes house mortgages as an example, attempts to interfere with
the evictions for non-payment of premiums on the ground that there
are young children in the home may well have the unintended consequence of restricting the availability of mortgage loans for families
with young children.

31 Crowe, 'Trolley full of empties', *The Guardian*, 8 August 1995.

32 See the report on the abandonment of the attempt by the international
community to impose sanctions on Kenya for failure to comply with
the UN Convention on Human Rights in *The Guardian*, 24 July 1995.

Chapter 8

A different world for children

In this final chapter I want to start by contrasting two very different approaches to the issue of improving the world for children. The first approach is that of 'demythologizing'. Once we know how people or society really work, proponents of this approach claim, we shall be able to identify those controls, the buttons and levers, that will enable social workers, judges and policy makers to steer people or society in one specified direction rather than another and, in the context of this book, that direction will be the one which improves children's lives. Depending on the circumstances, these controls could be technological, economic, psychological, legal, religious or political. They may involve such diverse techniques as, at one end of the spectrum, revealing the true power structure of society by removing the scales from people's eyes; and, at the other end, unmasking people and making the 'real self' or 'inner self' visible. For those concerned with the future of children they may include discovering how the family 'really functions' as a system, or getting behind the bright facade of advertising to reveal the poor nutritional value of 'junk foods'. It may also include placing hidden video cameras in a hospital ward in order to see whether a mother's account of her child's illness is true or whether it is she who is causing the child's symptoms. In the sociological and psychological literature one frequently finds the idea that progress can be achieved by revealing the shortcomings of 'self-serving truths', those widely held conceptions that people cling to, and exposing them for what they are. Indeed, opening our eyes to the misconceptions and ephemeral nature of much of what we accept as truth and reality is a very useful exercise. It is also, however, a misleading enterprise. It suggests that somewhere beyond the myths lies a universe called 'objective reality' or 'people as they really are' and that myth-destruction will provide us with a clear route to this world and these people. As an invitation to an ultimate deliverance from myth, these Enlightenment-inspired endeavours turn out to be no less mythical than the myths that their authors seek to destroy. The experience of the postmodernist and poststructuralist movement over the past two decades has taught us that there is no sustainable demarcation between myth and scientific correctness. It has been well-known since the time of Hegel that the very image that people maintain of themselves depends upon the identities available from the social environment in which they exist (Hegel, 1977). From this perspective, myths may be all we have, but this does not mean to say that all myths should be given equal status. There is no reason why different versions of society or different moral personae should not be compared and evaluated according to their benefits and shortcomings. The results of such comparisons and evaluations will differ according to the stance of the observer, but one thing they should not do is to transform the preferred identity into an absolute reality and make all others appear somehow false or phony. If certain preferred 'truths' later become mythical, that means that they were only 'true' for a certain time, space and cultural context in which they were predicated, which then fell into oblivion. They were also only true or mythical for those who shared the beliefs and commitments of the truth and myth claimers. Successful myths are those on which society comes to depend for its stability and continuity; they become unsuccessful when they are exposed as 'nothing more than myths'.

Where debunking myths takes on the form of an ideology, the holders of that ideology tend to believe that demythologizing will make it possible to put right what appears to have gone wrong with reality. Through exposure of the real world and people as they really are, the notion of reality on which the ideology depends will be seen as 'the truth'.

It would be as well for me to make it clear that, contrary to what some people may believe, neither I, as author of this book, nor Niklas Luhmann or the other theorists on whom I have drawn, would make any such claim for the theory of autopoiesis. Autopoiesis offers, not a belief system, but a description of society which presupposes the existence of innumerable other possible ways of describing society. It also accepts the fact that it too will be observed by other systems of knowledge and understanding which will inevitably reconstitute it within their epistemological framework. According to autopoietic theory, no one of these systems has the privilege of offering an exclusively correct view of society and no one of them is more 'mythical' than others.

Then there is a second approach which contrasts markedly with the first. This has been epitomized by the mysterious science fiction story with which Rex and Wendy Stainton Rogers open their book, *Stories of Childhood. Shifting Agendas of Child Concern*. This is 'The Tale of Nema'. Nema is a young woman who suddenly appears naked in the women's lavatories of a shopping mall at closing time. She seems to have totally lost her memory. Her appearance is of a girl of between 14 and 20 years old and on medical examination, it is found that Nema has borne a child. She remains silent about her past life and constructs an identity for herself from her experiences after her discovery in the lavatories. Various explanations are offered by the authors for her past and her present situation, but they conclude that 'Medical and social science . . . cannot give us an unambiguous answer, and neither can we reason one out from "common sense"'. They conclude that

> In the end we seem to be left with a moral decision – how to do what's right in a situation of uncertainty. . . . Do we turn to an 'expert' like a judge or psychiatrist? Or do we let Nema decide for herself? One solution favoured by moral philosophers would be to ask: who would I want making the decision if I were Nema? The usual answer is *me*, I would want to make that choice. But if Nema chose to be fourteen, would we see that as a sensible choice, or might we find ourselves thinking that anyone who made that choice wasn't rational enough to make it!
>
> (Stainton Rogers, 1992, p. 2, emphasis in original)

At last Nema herself relieves us of the dilemma, by blurting out that 'she is in fact a young woman social history student from the twenty-fourth century' (*ibid.*, p. 3). Her amnesia was hypnotically induced prior to her transportation back to our time. These facts were never supposed to emerge, but 'so bizarre did she find our world that her mind block failed. Now she cannot stop herself talking to her psychiatrist(!)'. 'Nema's narrative' reveals that

> Although age doesn't have the meaning in her society that it does in ours, Nema is in fact thirteen. Changes in environmental conditions, diet and health care mean that most young people reach full reproductive sexual maturity at around the age of ten. In her world, quite a lot of young people decide to have children in

their early teens, as they are by then physically capable and economically and socially independent.

(ibid., p. 3)

In Nema's world there is no minimum age for driving or for working. 'Clever' cars which can sense hazards mean that children of
three or four can safely go out alone. Advances in the technologies
of teaching and learning mean that 'by around seven most young
people can run their lives more or less independently from adults'
(ibid., p. 4). By the age of seven or eight people had a wide network
of friends who would move from one person's home to another as a
'gang'. Loyalty and mutual support to one's 'gang', rather than
'olders' was the norm. 'Gangs' were places to experiment with interpersonal and sexual relationships.

> There was 'no age of consent' as such; any 'competent' had the right
> to 'body control' over sex as over anything else. 'Olders' had little to
> do with the young and little power over them – one result was that
> physical and sexual abuse across age was virtually unknown.
>
> (ibid., p. 4)

The Stainton Rogers use Nema's tale first to challenge 'the idea that
childhood is "a thing" that can be known and defined objectively'
(ibid., p. 5). They argue that 'every story gains its meaning through
a socially sedimented "contract" for engaging our regard. . . . The
reader is drawn into a social process between peruser and perused'
(ibid., p. 6). Second, they want to challenge the idea that there are
such things as real 'facts' or a 'true knowledge' where ideas about
children's welfare are concerned. The 'fact', they argue,

> that child prostitutes and some sexually abused children (as does
> Nema) show 'precocious' sexual development' can only be dis-
> covered within certain social regards, in which there is a pre-
> scribed appropriate or normal age to be a thing called sexual.
>
> (ibid., p. 6)

The basic thesis of their book, then, is that 'we live in a world which
is produced through stories' (ibid., p. 6). So far as children are concerned, they

> are drawn into this web of understanding (and their material
> consequences) from the moment (. . .) whenever they enter the
> social world. Our stories of childhood largely pre-date and create
> the locations in the social world for each child. . . . All this gives

the term 'story' a much broader span than does its day-to-day definition.

(ibid., p. 7)

What does this story tell the readers of the Stainton Rogers' book? Clearly it challenges the very concept of childhood as something fixed and unchanging. Instead childhood appears as a free-floating notion, the interpretation of which depends upon the particular culture in which it appears (Ariès, 1962). There are clearly points of contact between the approach of the Stainton Rogers and the theoretical orientation of my book. In reading the problems facing moral campaigns to improve the world for children, readers of this book will also have found themselves drawn into the uncomfortable situation of being both 'peruser and perused', observer and observed. You start by wanting to strip away the myths, but find yourselves stripping away all certainties, by seeing your own beliefs as to what is right or wrong for children and society as being no more objectively correct or true than the myths that you have so effectively destroyed. How will you know if you have created a better or worse world for children? Asking children at some future time cannot give you the answer. Asking today's children at a future date, when they are adults, will tell you only how those adults see their childhood and compare their childhood with that of other children. Can you with any confidence claim that the lives of children today are better or worse than children who lived two hundred years ago? They are certainly different, but as Nema's tale reveals, the expectations of childhood and the way that we evaluate the 'quality of life' have changed in all kinds of ways.

CONSTRUCTIONS OF HAPPINESS, HARM AND SUFFERING

In this book I have deliberately turned my back on the bleak forecasts of media pundits concerning children and their future, with their view of modern society in a state of major moral crisis with families disintegrating and children out of control, using drugs, sleeping on the streets and committing crimes. I have also put to one side the major themes that appear to preoccupy policy makers and writers on social policy – the vision of a pluralist and multi-cultural world where, it is argued, moral principles have become relative and uncertain, leading to a multitude of often incommensurable and conflicting values and beliefs and a rise of nationalist movements and fundamentalist religions, and so of simple reassuring solutions. The message that seems to emerge from both these kinds of analysis of the social situation is that the only sure way forward is for each person to steer his or her own path towards a personal salvation and a better personal future. According to this view, in a chaotic world in which there are no fixed points, it is up to the individual to develop his or her own fixed points. But, as the explorations that I have undertaken in the pages of this book have shown, this is hardly a solution for children, whose only points of knowledge and understanding of the world are those fixed for them in advance. Children are beings outside ourselves, but beings for whom we feel ourselves to be responsible. It is in the context of such pessimistic and individualistic perspectives, precisely as an acknowledgement of this responsibility and of the existence of an uncertain present and a future existing beyond our own lives, that moral agendas are drawn up and moral campaigns mounted to protect children from suffering, and to create a better, less harmful, world for them.

Some harms and suffering, it is true, are universal and timeless. Sickness, serious physical injury, malnutrition, and bereavement of a parent almost by definition give rise to suffering among children and adults alike. Reducing and controlling, and campaigns to eliminate the sources of such suffering, have always been tasks for society, even if the methods of achieving such objectives have often resulted in harm and suffering to others (who were once seen as excluded from society). Where such control has not been possible, society has always found ways of explaining harm to and the suffering of children in ways which make it more acceptable. But today's moral campaigns go far beyond these aspirations. What then has changed?

What has changed in modern society is, first, the impossibility of attributing harms to children to sources external to society. As I have already discussed (Chapter 5), it is no longer possible to maintain an explanatory account of social events which points to God or the devil as being the source of harm and suffering. Nor is it acceptable to designate enemies as 'forces of darkness' as if they existed outside the boundaries of society. What we have to acknowledge today is that even enemies are part of modern society, which is world society. The havoc they inflict is seen as the results of decisions, of risks unscrupulously or ill-advisedly taken.

Second, what has changed is the increased specificity of the targets of moral campaigns. While wars, famines, disease and natural disasters may still be matters of grave concern to society, these are seen as demanding political, diplomatic, medical, military or economic responses. These campaigns against 'enemies' do not specifically concern children, but relate to the precise nature of the 'disaster' and the 'human suffering' caused. Those campaigns directed specifically at children, on the other hand, are rooted in the principles of moral philosophy – the proper treatment of the weak and defenceless, the protection of the innocent, the acknowledgement of rights to those who are unable to challenge decisions made for their welfare. Moral campaigns today which take an ideological stance for and on behalf of a better future for children tend to select as their targets harms which they identify (rightly or wrongly) as very specific to children.

The combination of these two developments has made it possible to mobilize people in national and global campaigns for child protection and the promotion of children's rights. A belief that *rights are right* and cannot be wrong, justifies the essential rightness of attempts to impose children's rights upon nation states and the decision making operations of organizations. Children's rights, according to this agenda, cannot do otherwise than promote children's interests. Conversely the ills and harms to children are seen as the result of human error, ignorance or perversity resulting from a failure to respect or take sufficient account of children's rights. As such these failures may, it is believed, be rectified by obliging, persuading or educating people, organizations and nation states to act in different ways.

It is at this point that morality appears to confront relativism, for in order for these moral agendas to be adopted and for these moral campaigns to succeed there has to be a consensus or unity around what constitutes benefits or harms for children or good or bad behaviour towards them. According to this view, the regulation of harms can only be conducted along ideological lines. One group has to prove that its identification of harms and their causes are right and alternative notions of harm and their causes, wrong. The result of such campaigns has been to create a series of social 'catastrophes' all of which revolve around highly specific harms to children – child-battering, sexual abuse, truanting, educational failure, drug-abuse, bullying, juvenile crime, etc. At times these have degenerated into a form of ideological warfare which rages around the extent of the problem, its causes and ways of controlling it. Child sexual abuse and juvenile delinquency are the two obvious examples, where gender politics and party politics have taken up cudgels to fight for different accounts of the causes and different ways of limiting the effects. These wars may rage between different belligerent parties, depending on the issue, yet always without ever resolving the question of which of the moral agendas was right and which wrong. Nevertheless, they can be seen as reiterating and reinforcing the message that it is possible both to identify 'rightness' and 'wrongness' in these situations and, once these two sides have been identified, to put into operation a series of measures, based on one or other version or on a compromise between the two, which will be effective in regulating the situation. The point that I want now to make and that I have emphasized throughout this book is that the effectiveness of such measures can never be guaranteed by either or any of these competing moral agendas. Indeed, the eventual form of the measures taken will remove them from the sphere of morality to be determined, not by the victors in the ideological contest, but by the authoritative pronouncements emerging from society's authority discourses, the communications of those of society's systems which society has designated as sites of authority.

What one is left with, therefore, is, at one level, a text or discourse which concerns itself with harms and suffering to children and applies a set of values and principles supposedly capable of ending such harms and suffering to children. Simultaneously, at another level, there exists a network of social systems, which are blind to moral values and principles and which can deal with harms and sufferings only in the narrow terms in which each of these systems is able to make sense of its environment. Both these ways of representing 'the state of things' are deployed quite independently of one another. These two levels operate in parallel, the one being capable of producing only irritations or perturbations for the other. The dilemma of dealing with the aspirations of regulation in modern society, therefore, is the result of the unbridged, and seemingly unbridgeable gap, between these two levels.

THE LIMITS OF MORAL AGENDAS FOR CHILDREN

Bearing this in mind, let us look for one last time at the global distinction that is at the root of and informs all regulatory measures concerning children. This is that children are fundamentally different from adults. In the contemporary world it is this distinction that gives meaning to and allows specifically moral agendas for and on behalf of children to separate themselves from the generality of moral values and principles. It finds expression, as we have seen, in two seemingly contradictory regulatory norms. The one seeks to protect children and promote their welfare through paternalistic measures while the other seeks to grant them a degree of autonomy. What may have appeared paradoxical for moral philosophers re-emerges within regulatory instruments, such as the United Nations Convention, as not merely commensurable, but even as mutually enhancing principles, for both succeed in designating children as essentially different from adults. Children's rights are not the same as those of adults; they come with a label which specifically defines them as applying only to children. In granting rights to children, therefore, regulatory bodies, while recognizing children as citizens, are at the same time emphasizing the difference between them and adults (see pages 169-170).

Why should so much significance be placed today on the difference that children represent? There are various answers and various kinds of answers to this question. One answer of a general nature is that this representation of children should be seen in the context of the uncertainty of contemporary life and, in particular, in the fragility of families in post-industrial countries which, it is argued, has given an unprecedented symbolic significance to children. For a number of reasons, children appear to give meaning to people's lives today in ways and to a degree that is probably unprecedented. To quote Ulrich Beck again, 'the child is the source of the last remaining, irrevocable, unchangeable primary relationship' (Beck, 1992 p. 118). They serve to anchor adults emotionally in a fluctuating and unreliable world. Although children, as individuals, are of course in a constant state of change, they have come in some paradoxical way, through their perceived vulnerability and dependence, to represent something constant, permanent and unchanging – something to heap affection upon, something to be responsible for, something to be protected, something to be fought over, but above all something to be understood and explained. David Archard remarks,

> it is important to note how extensive and sophisticated is the knowledge that we in the twentieth century can claim to have of the child's nature, and how this knowledge turns on an appreciation of childhood *as an abstraction from the particularities of children*. What the present age knows all about is what it is to be at the stage of and in the state of childhood.
>
> (Archard, 1993, p. 30, emphasis added)

What is also important to note, however, is that these 'abstractions from the particularities of childhood' are not *facts* about childhood but beliefs which serve as certainties to hold together particular ideological accounts of what the world is now and what it could be. Again, what the present age knows about are not *facts* about the state and stages of childhood, but particular accounts that carry with them a seal of authority. These accounts often conflict with the images and practices towards children favoured within particular cultural settings which rely upon different certainties and different abstractions, so that the identification of one abstraction rests on one set of particularities or partial account of what children are and could become. It is hardly surprising that Jo Boydon should complain that in some respects, 'the move to set global standards for childhood and common policies for child welfare may be far from the enlightened step anticipated by its proponents' (Boydon, 1990, p. 208; also see Chapter 7).

Yet where do these apparent global standards, this knowledge both about the state and stages of childhood and what should be done to meet children's needs, come from? They are 'facts' because and only because modern society recognizes them as factual, just as Nema's society of the twenty-fourth century recognized a very different set of 'facts' as factual. On examination, however, it is clear that these abstractions which we treat as factual conform to the positive expectations generated by those institutions that have evolved to provide clarity and certainty in social relations. They are rooted in the knowledge and understandings of those functionally differentiated systems, the sites that society has selected for its authoritative accounts of causality and its agendas for the future. As we have seen, it is the programmes of systems such as law, science, politics and economics, which provide the formal decision making organizations in society with the knowledge and criteria on the basis of which they are able to operate.

We are left then with the situation where the moral agendas for the creation of a better world for children reiterate the positive values of each of society's function systems: truth and health for science, justice for law, equality for politics and wealth for economics. (One could also add progress through knowledge for education.) Each of these values serves as a generalized medium of communication, providing society with the belief that the achievement of these desirable goals are possible for children and for the future, but also that they are possible through the operation of the existing institutions that maintain the beliefs as their positive values and as ideals capable of realization. The problem, however, is that while these values may represent goals to be pursued by social institutions, they are only idealizations. The daily operation of these systems is concerned, as we have seen, not with putting into effect moral agendas, but with transforming events that occur in its environment into knowledge that can then be productive of facts, decisions, statements and results, etc., upon which other social systems and the society as a whole are able to rely.

While justice may represent the ideal for law, law's programmes cannot distinguish what is just from what is not just, for the simple reason that any agreement about what is actually just or unjust in a particular case is extremely unlikely and so such a thing as certainty will not be available from any attempt to distinguish between the two. What law is able to do is to decide with certainty what is lawful and what unlawful. In the same way science has no way of producing statements of absolute truth, but is able to determine which statements are scientifically correct and which are false. The political system offers, not equality, but the distinction between government and opposition; economics offers, not wealth, but the distinction of profit and loss; the education system, not progress through knowledge, but the distinction of pass/fail. Each on its own terms and in its own specific way offers certainty, but this is not certainty linked to any idea of progress or the dissemination and promotion of moral values.

At the same time, morality and those belief systems which depend upon moral programmes are necessarily blind to this distinction between generalized ideal values and system communications. For them, either the two are identical or the latter are seen as nothing other than obstructions to the former, the 'practical problems', which I discussed in Chapter 1 as factors which appear to block the path to progress. Yet to an observer of social systems, it is no surprise that the notion of children's rights within politics, for example, comes to be seen simultaneously as the route to a fairer, safer, more equal world (and as the imposition of unacceptable demands by foreign powers); or within law as legal authorities to be deployed in order to win one's case (and to be resisted in order not to lose one's case); or within economics as opportunities for lawyers to increase their earnings (and as a heavy financial burden for carpet manufacturers employing children at low wages). Seen from the perspective of an observer of social systems, the problem for would-be constructors of a better world for children is not that which moral campaigns would have us believe, but those to which morality is blind, for morality cannot see beyond the moral ideals which social institutions represent, but which they have such difficulty in achieving. It cannot peer into the black boxes to observe the amoral operations of these organizations. It is able only to interpret as *immorality* (the negative side of the distinction of morals) the *amorality* of social systems, which are obliged to behave in ways that are beyond good and evil or, in Luhmann's terms, to do only what they do. From the perspective of morality, the immorality of systems needs to be subjected to suitable remedial measures, but for each of the systems being observed, they are only doing their job.

This is close to the point which I made in Chapter 1 – the confusion within moral agendas between consciousness and society, when it came to tackling social issues. What I would now wish to add to this earlier point is the idea that moral belief systems have no other way to promulgate their social message than through partial, idealized visions of social behaviour and of what constitutes society. For them to see the social world in any other way would be to lose hold of the ability to distinguish between what is good for children and what is bad for children, which provides such belief systems with their moral identity. For them there is no alternative.

In a similar way, science, law, politics and all other social authority systems have no alternative but to proceed *as if their version of reality, their internally-generated account of the social world were true*. In practice, however, the truth about society that each one of them generates depends upon its ability to reconstitute other 'truths' generated and communicated by other systems. Systems, unfortunately, do not share their particular self-image. Each is obliged to communicate by reconstructing that system as part of its own environment in its own idiosyncratic terms.

THE IDEAL OF REGULATION

The difficulty that autopoietic observers are able to recognize with the claims of those who would regulate harmful behaviour to children concerns the restricted vision of those social systems which are obliged to put into effect the regulatory measures. Each of these systems is programmed to see itself as capable of recognizing a problem, but 'the problem' that they are able to recognize is necessarily formulated in terms that make it appear as if successful regulation of the problem by that system is a strong probability.

The achievement of the children's rights movement in obtaining so many signatories to the United Nations Convention may, for example, be regarded as a solution generated by international politics to the problem of children's helplessness and suffering. Politics, however, is one and only one social system. Just as it is apparent to those who observe the political system that the success of political parties in democracies depends upon them selling their vision of the future to the electorate, it is also clear that politicians have no choice but to make it appear that the world is organized in such a way as to allow for the possibility that their policies might succeed. This is necessarily a simplified version of society and the world and an optimistic account of the ways in which the desired goals may be attained. Moreover, the same political programme also requires the same politicians to account for failure in ways that make it appear that *success is still a possibility*. As one commentator recently remarked on the subject of political regulation:

> State failure encourages people to think that more laws, taxes, regulators and inspectors are needed to ensure success. In case of market failure, people resort instinctively to the alternative remedy of the state. But in cases of state failure, nobody questions whether there are limits beyond which the state ceases to be effective. Instead, the failure is plugged with a new regulation.
>
> (Hobson 1995, p. 10)

What autopoietic systems theory tells us, and what this commentator omits to emphasize, however, is that within politics the limits of effective regulation are defined by politics and only by politics in ways that see law and fiscal controls as nothing other than instruments of 'the state' for the achievement of political ends. If they work for a time in giving the impression that the state or government is able to control the problem, then they are recognized as politically effective. By using other, non-political criteria of effectiveness, be they legal, moral, religious, economic or scientific, an external observer of politics may demonstrate that politically effective is not the same as lawful, morally right, in accordance with God's laws, cost-effective or scientifically valid. This leads to the paradoxical situation where the observer of politics realizes, on the one hand, that success or failure in the regulation of conduct towards children is possible only at the price of politics ignoring complexity, but, on the other hand, recognizes that any satisfactory analysis of how or why regulation works or does not work depends explicitly upon the recognition of the same complexity.

Where do we go from here? If the regulating system is able to judge its own regulatory efforts only on its own terms, and must invariably reconstruct external reports of effectiveness in ways that make sense to those terms, what hope is there of defining and controlling harms to children through the existing social institutions? Gunther Teubner in a recent talk suggested that law should switch its role from that of balancing a pluralism of interests to that of balancing a pluralism of discourses (Teubner, in press). It is law that would then take on the task of determining how children's welfare should be defined and what social system should be employed in what context to regulate behaviour towards children, and what criteria of success should be applied. Presumably, therefore, where the health of certain groups of children in a developing country was causing concern, the legal system would decide whether more money was needed and whether government policies on overseas aid should be altered. At the very least, the law should be in a position to limit the damage caused by one system's operations on other systems engaged in dealing with the problem. It should be in a position, therefore, to order warring states to allow relief convoys to enter the area so that medical supplies might be distributed for the benefit of sick children. But how does law know such things, except in terms of its own lawful/unlawful coding? We seem to be back in the utopian world of a universal legal order, where decisions of international or constitutional courts are regarded universally as supreme authorization on what is right and wrong for children.

If one applies Teubner's formula to the protection of children against abuse within families, it may be possible to see how the legal system might determine, for example, to what extent medical evidence should be admissible or whether gender or race differences or social factors, such as poverty or unemployment, should be taken into account in the decision making process. Indeed, the law at present already performs some of these tasks, but in accepting them it exposes itself to accusations that it is guilty of causing damage not only to children, but also to other systems, which are also in the business of determining what is and is not in the best interests of children.[1]

At least, it could be argued, Teubner has helped to change the question from 'How do we create a better world for children?' to 'How can we arrive at the most socially acceptable way of determining what is good or bad for children?'. While this second, replacement question is answerable only by stepping outside the boundaries of one particular social system, the original question is answerable only by remaining firmly within those boundaries.

The other solution proposed by Gunther Teubner to deal with this clash of discourses is for law to lend its authority to external autonomous systems, constituting them in ways which allow them to reach their own decisions, recognized as 'legally valid' by law. Indeed, we have already experienced a trend in this direction with the introduction of mediation, alternative dispute resolution projects and family group conferences and meetings. One can link this solution with Niklas Luhmann's enthusiasm for 'system planning' which I discussed in Chapter 6. New situations should attract systemic analyses rather than the usual accounts of interests and actions, but they should also be treated as an opportunity for the creation of new autonomous systems with authority to regulate the situation, taking into account its specific features, including the clash or potential clash of discourses or system-specific validations.

Much depends on the capacity for creativity and innovation. To some degree the fragmentation of modern society allows space for new developments in ways which would not have been possible in traditional or pre-modern societies. On the other hand, the lack of any overriding authority produces many false starts – embryo regulatory systems which fail to regulate, child abuse controls which prove to be themselves abusive to children.

Social regulation is not simply a matter of devising new means of control; it may also involve the relaxing of controls. Individuals, pairs of individuals, families and small communities may up to a point be permitted to select their own forms of internal regulation, without the need for social system authority. They may, if they want, choose a humanist moral code, the words of Muhammad, interpretations of the unconscious or the position of the planets, to guide their behaviour. This freedom of choice, as we have seen, cannot exist where the belief abounds that there is authority to subject all forms of harmful behaviour to children to effective state or intergovernmental controls. Teubner's second solution, that of delegating authority, in theory allows these choices to be made in areas of activity which were previously allocated to society's function systems as falling within their sphere of authority.

One way of avoiding these problems is to avoid direct regulation altogether. It is possible, for instance, for organizations to decide not to make decisions in future, but rather to allow situations to evolve in ways that will allow people to find their own solutions to their problems. Mediation is an example. Here, the regulatory system attempts to reformulate conflicts in ways which allow the disputants themselves to arrive at a solution. This solution may theoretically draw upon the shared values of the individuals in conflict, whether or not such values correspond to the normative expectations of those social function systems which society has designated as authoritative. In practice, these normative expectations are not so easy to avoid, particularly where the possibility exists for either party to refer the matter to law or to use economic power in the event of no solution being agreed.

Of course, the very act of identifying problems and deciding what does and what does not need a decision may be seen as an indirect form of regulation. Even if the precise form of the steps to be taken is left for others to decide, it is the problem-identifier who has defined the issues and set the limits, if not the agenda, for the problem's solution.

Although it may also be possible for a system to renounce totally the authority to regulate in certain situations, in practice, however, this usually means leaving the way clear for other social systems to impose their own agendas. Despite the political rhetoric, 'market forces' do not represent total liberty from controls, but the substitution of economic rationality for other forms of regulation. Likewise, alternative dispute resolution processes to the courts, rarely mean freedom from any form of regulatory control, but rather the substitution of distinctions such as helpful/unhelpful, good for children/bad for children, conflictual/cooperative, for lawful/unlawful. In these cases what appears to have happened is that government or courts have decided not to continue to be held accountable for losses or failures, no longer to be the risk takers.

A similar situation exists when the problem is passed from one system to another. While at the level of interpersonal relations it is possible to invoke personal belief systems to justify and legitimate decisions, at the social level decisions have to be constructed in ways that have meaning for society. Harms to children, once identified within a system which society vests with authority, tend to be regarded, in a sense, as the responsibility and the property of that system. From that time onwards measures aimed at protection against and avoidance of these harms have to conform to system assessments of what constitutes risk to children and of what measures may be taken to prevent harm. The system, being closed, is blind to the damage that it may be causing to the integrity of other systems. From the perspective of science, for example, law may appear to distort and simplify to the point of absurdity the knowledge of the psychiatric and psychological sciences by reconstructing them as 'expert evidence' (Wynne, 1989; King and Piper, 1995). Similarly, law may see science as disregarding justice and fairness in its procedures for obtaining and testing 'the truth'.

THE LIMITS OF SOLIDARITY AND COOPERATION

For some observers of society 'real change' may only be possible through violent revolution or some massive upheaval in the way that society is organized. Yet the version of society that I have relied upon throughout this book does not preclude such future possibilities. It does not prescribe the kind of political or economic arrangements that might be thought to be necessary in the future for achieving the goal of 'making things better for children'. Most of these revolutionary accounts tend to assume, perhaps idealistically, that this goal is achievable *through the concerted efforts of people*, whether they be Muslims, Marxists, fundamentalist Christians, socialists, or communitarians. The essential point is that the achievement of order and stability, justice and prosperity, holiness, health and happiness, is seen as being firmly in the hands of people whose conscious acts to change the world will bring about this better future. Success in putting into effect projects for the future of society, whether the product of a political consensus, moral majority or revolutionary council, or whether revealed in a party manifesto or a utopian dream, depend first upon winning people's support for a particular ideological agenda.

Second, success relies upon the formulation of ways of harnessing people's energy and creativity so that they promote and serve these projects and the values that they represent. This essentially is a notion of a future society which, unlike the present one, is capable of being regulated in ways that promote children's interests. Yet just like the conceptions of the present society which have evolved within moral philosophy, it sees people, their consciousness and that consciousness translated directly into behaviour, either individual or collective, as the key to a better future.

I have at no point in this book questioned the belief that people are able to work together to combat such problems as child abuse and the exploitation of children. This is not in dispute. Nor have I raised any doubts over the notion that within institutional settings lawyers and psychologists, scientists and politicians, economists and medical experts are capable of cooperation. The problems with which this book has been concerned do not arise from such inter-personal behaviour (although it may well relate to the possibilities for understanding such behaviour). These problems arises rather at the level of social systems of communication. It is that these sys-tems are able to relate to one another only by attempting to impose their own self-generated evaluations and criteria for success upon the other. From within each system this may give the impression of success or at least give rise to the belief that success is possible, but from outside the system this impression is likely to appear as illuso-ry, or even as the 'enslavement' of one system by another. In either case, what may appear to fulfil the ideals of cooperation and coor-dination on closer examination reveals some confusion. People who by designation are identified with one scheme of interpretation and knowledge are in practice relying upon a very different scheme. Policemen may be operating as social workers, social workers as policemen, judges as psychiatrists, psychiatrists as judges. Alternatively, the same people may be shifting from one interpretive scheme to another without warning and without clarity as to the criteria which authorizes such switching to take place.[2]

WHAT IS TO BE DONE?

You cannot assess the value of economic explanations on religious criteria or use law to judge between scientific theories. It is no less impossible for the sociological observer to evaluate those many and varied agendas for making the world a better place for children. Only by ceasing to observe sociologically would such judgments be possible. As a 'conscious system' it would be quite possible for me to change perspectives and, at the last moment, switch to some dif-ferent perspective, some *modus operandi* that would enable me to compare the various proposals on the basis of their likely ability to meet children's needs, cost effectiveness, fairness, morality, respect for traditional values, promotion of child autonomy. This would leave the way clear for critics to locate my position on whatever spectrum of beliefs and values that happened to appeal to them and to evaluate all the preceding pages of the book from this revelation of my 'true colours'. There will doubtless be some critics who will attempt this exercise in any event, because for them there is perhaps no other way of making sense of a book which purports to be about children and their interests.

If this book is to 'make sense' in the way that I intended when writing it, then any criticisms of its substance should respect the serious attempt I have made to remove myself from all the ongoing debates about children's rights, their needs and their interests, and all the discussions about the ways of promoting them and regulating and controlling the behaviour of adults so as to ensure respect and regard for them. Criticism should be concerned primarily with the version of society and the hermeneutic device of social function systems that I have applied to these issues. It should concentrate on the value or otherwise of this analysis in constructing a theoretical model which goes beyond the existing ways of seeing society and the efforts to guarantee a better future society for children. My sociological observations can and should, of course, be subjected to such sociological scrutiny.

Any final conclusions on my part will, therefore, be restricted to a brief summary of what I see as being the advantageous features of a sociological perspective which sees the world as a society of communications organized according to social systems. These are:

1 A clear distinction between the motivations, aspirations and beliefs of people and the operations of social systems. The one may involve moral principles, faith, values and ideologies, the other is concerned with disembodied, mechanistic operations going about their business of making things happen, so that it is possible that other things may happen and society can continue to exist. They do what they do, no more and no less.

2 A modesty as to what is possible for sociology and sociologists to achieve. This involves a total renunciation of any ambition to solve the world's problems or even a small part of those problems. The only way it is possible for sociologists to act as if they are capable of changing the world by direct action is by entering into those discourses and debates constructed within political, educational, scientific, legal, moral or other domains. As soon as they do this, they cease to be sociologists and lose the capacity for sociological observation. This is not intended as a puritan or ascetic code of discipline for sociologists, but merely as an observation that once sociologists see society as an entity that can be changed by wilful behaviour, they will have reconstructed society

in a way that ignores fundamental obstacles to change in one direction rather than another, and confused what seems desirable with what seems possible.

3   A clear recognition of the impossibility of direct communication between systems and, in particular, between morality and social systems and between those social systems which society has designated as the sites of authoritative accounts. This phenomenon of system non-communication provides the language for a description of society which acknowledges the existence of different perspectives, different codes of interpretation, different bodies of knowledge and different criteria for evaluation. It may also reflect some of the frustration and impotence that those who work towards 'making things better' must feel.

4   The acceptance that, so far as changing society is concerned, irritants (or perturbations) are the most that any system, whether conscious or social, can achieve. But even this may be quite an achievement. This acceptance involves the recognition that social consequences, both intended and unintended, are contingent not on high motivation, thorough research or careful planning (although all of these may affect the ways in which the irritant is perceived), but upon the ways in which each system reconstitutes the irritating event occurring in its environment. From this point on, social consequences will depend upon the way in which other systems themselves respond to the secondary irritant caused by that system's response. While all of this may lead to exciting and complex accounts of causes and effects, it does nothing to help the task of predicting the future except perhaps by convincing would-be prophets that the future is unpredictable.

It is of course possible that the sociological reformulations I have attempted in this book will act as irritants to some systems and that these systems will in time respond to them. Indeed, it is also possible that some of their reactions will improve the lives of and create a better world for some children. But there can, of course, be no guarantee that this will happen!

NOTES

1   See King and Trowell (1993).
2   See the discussion of the effects of the Children Act of 1989 in King and Trowell (1992).

Bibliography and further reading

CHAPTER 1 GOOD INTENTIONS INTO SOCIAL ACTION

Archard, D. (1993) *Children, Rights and Childhood*, London: Routledge.
Beck, U. (1992) *Risk Society*, London: Sage.
Flew, A. (ed.) (1979) *A Dictionary of Philosophy*, London: Pan.
Foerster, H. von (1981) *Observing Systems*, Seaside, Cal.: Intersystems Publications.
Foucault, M. (1979) *The History of Sexuality, Vol III: The Case of the Self*, New York: Pantheon.
Howitt, D. (1992) *Child Abuse Errors. When Good Intentions go Wrong*, Hemel Hempstead: Harvester-Wheatsheaf.
King, M. (1993) 'The "Truth" about Autopoiesis' *Journal of Law and Society*, 20(2): p. 1.
King, M. and Schütz, A. (1994) 'The Ambitious Modesty of Niklas Luhmann' *Journal of Law and Society*, 21(3): p. 261.
Luhmann, N. (1990) *Essays on Self Reference*, New York: Columbia University Press.
—— (1986) 'The Autopoiesis of Social Systems' in F. Geyer and J. van der Zouwen (eds) *Sociocybernetic Paradoxes: Observation, Control and Evolution of Self-Steering Systems*, London: Sage
—— (1987) 'The Representation of Society within Society' *Current Sociology*, 35: p. 101.
—— (1988a) 'Closure and Openness: On the Reality in the World of Law' in G. Teubner (ed.) *Autopoietic Law. A New Approach to Law and Society*, Berlin and New York: Walter de Gruyter.
—— (1988b) 'Familiarity, Confidence and Trust: Problems and Alternatives' in D. Gambetta (ed.) *Gambetta Trust*, Cambridge: Cambridge University Press.
—— (1988c) 'The Sociological Observations of the Theory and Practice of Law' in A. Febbrajo (ed.) *European Yearbook of the Sociology of Law*, Milan: Giuffrè.
—— (1988d) 'Tautology and Paradox in the Self-Description of Modern Society' *Sociological Theory*, 6: p. 21.
—— (1988e) 'The Third Question: The Creative Use of Paradox in Law and Legal History' *Journal of Law and Society*, 15: p. 153.

—— (1988f) 'The Unity of the Legal System' in G. Teubner (ed.) *Autopoietic Law: A New Approach to Law and Society*, Berlin and New York: Walter de Gruyter.

—— (1989a) *Ecological Communications*, Oxford: Polity.

—— (1989b) 'Law as a Social System' *Northwestern University Law Review*, 83(1& 2): p. 136.

—— (1990a) 'The Coding of the Legal System' in A. Febbrajo and G. Teubner (eds) *State, Law, Economy as Autopoietic Systems*, Milan: Giuffrè.

—— (1990b) 'The Cognitive Program of Constructivism and a Reality that Remains Unknown' in W. Krohn, G. Kuppers and H. Nowotny (eds) *Self-Organization, Portrait of a Scientific Revolution. Sociology of the Sciences Yearbook*, Dordrecht: Kluwer.

—— (1990c) *Essays on Self Reference*, New York: Columbia University Press.

—— (1990d) *Political Theory in the Welfare State*, Berlin and New York: Walter de Gruyter.

—— (1992a) 'Operational Closure and Structural Coupling: The Differentiation of the Legal System' *Cardozo Law Review*, 13: p. 1419.

—— (1992b) 'Some Problems with "Reflexive Law"' in G. Teubner and A. Febbrajo (eds) *European Yearbook of the Sociology of Law*, Milan: Giuffrè.

—— (1993a) 'The Code of the Moral' *Cardozo Law Review*, 14: p. 995.

—— (1993b) *Risk: A Sociological Theory*, New York: Aldine de Gruyter.

—— (1995) 'Legal Argumentation: An Analysis of its Form' *Modern Law Review*, 58: p. 285.

—— (1995b) Social Systems, (trans) J. Bednartz Jr. Stanford U.S.A.: Stanford Universtiy Press.

Murphy, W. T. (1984) 'Modern Times. Niklas Luhmann on Law Politics and Social Theory' *Modern Law Review*, 47: p. 603.

—— (1994) 'Systems of Systems: Some Issues in the Relationship between Law and Autopoiesis' *Law and Critique*, v: p. 241.

Nelken, D. (1988) 'Changing Paradigms in the Sociology of Law' in G. Teubner (ed.) *Autopoietic Law: A New Approach to Law and Society*, Berlin and New York: Walter de Gruyter.

Rottleuthner, H. (1989) 'A Purified Sociology of Law: Niklas Luhmann on the Autonomy of the Legal System' *Law and Society Review*, 23: p. 779.

Sciulli, D. (1994) 'An Interview with Niklas Luhmann' *Theory, Culture and Society*, 11: p. 37.

Stainton Rogers, R. and W. (1992) *Stories of Childhood. Shifting Agendas of Child Concern*, Hemel Hempstead, Herts: Harvester-Wheatsheaf.

Teubner, G. (1989) 'How the Law Thinks: Toward a Constructivist Epistomology of Law' *Law and Society Review*, 23: p. 727.

—— (1993) *Law as an Autopoietic System*, Oxford: Blackwell.

CHAPTER 2 CHILD ABUSE AND THE REGULATION OF MALE POWER

Archard, D. (1993) *Children, Rights and Childhood*, London: Routledge.

Astor, H. (1991) *Position Paper on Mediation*, National Committee on Violence against Women.

Bayer, T. and Conners, R. (1988) 'The Emergence of Child Sexual Abuse from the Shadow of Sexism' *Response*, p. 12.

Blackburn, K. and Tooze, B. (1994) 'Narcissism and Self-Image in Male–Female Abuse' *Probation Journal*, 41(2): pp. 66–72.

Calhoun, C. (1994) 'Social Theory and the Politics of Identity' in C. Calhoun (ed.) *Social Theory and the Politics of Identity*, Oxford: Blackwell.

Dominelli, L. (1986) 'Father–daughter Incest: Patriarchy's Shameful Secret' *Critical Social Policy*, 6(16).

Dominelli, L. and MacLoed, E. (1989) *Feminist Social Work*, London: Macmillan.

Festinger, L. (1964) *When Prophesy Fails: A Social and Psychological Study of a Modern Group that Predicted the Destruction of the World*, New York: Harper and Row.

Fischer, K., Vidmar, N. and Rene, E. (1993) 'The Culture of Battering and the Role of Mediation in Domestic Violence Cases' *Southern Methodist University Law Review*, 46: p. 2117.

Gordon, L. (1988a) *Heroes of their own Lives: The Politics and History of Family Violence, Boston 1880–1960*, London: Virago.

—— (1988b) 'The Politics of Child Sexual Abuse: Notes from American History' *Feminist Review*, 28: p. 56.

Hanmer, J., Radford, J. and Stanko, E. A. (1989) *Women, Policing and Male Violence*, London: Routledge.

Herman, D. (1993) 'Review of "Understanding Sexual Violence: A Study of Convicted Rapists" by Diana Scully' *Social and Legal Studies*, 2: p. 239.

Kelly, L. (1988) 'What's in a Name? Defining Child Sexual Abuse' *Feminist Review*, 28: p. 65.

King, M. and Piper, C. (1995) *How the Law Thinks about Children* (2nd edn), Aldershot, Hants: Arena.

King, M. and Trowell, J. (1992) *Children's Welfare and the Law: The Limits of Legal Intervention*, London: Sage.

Kirsta, A. (1994) *Deadlier than the Male: Violence and Aggression in Women*, London: HarperCollins.

Lorenz, E. (1964) 'The Problem of Deducing the Climate from the Governing Equation' *Tellus*, 16: p. 1.

Luhmann, N. (1990) *Essays on Self Reference* (Chapter 7), New York: Columbia University Press.

MacKinnon, C. A. (1989) *Toward a Feminist Theory of the State*, Cambridge, Mass. and London: Harvard University Press.

MacLoed, M. and Saraga, E. (1988) 'Challenging the Orthodoxy: Towards a Feminist Theory and Practice' *Feminist Review*, 28: p 16.

Mahoney, M. (1991) 'Legal Images of Battered Women: Redefining the Issue of Separation' *Michigan Law Review*, 90: p. 2.

Manning, N. (1985) 'Constructing Social Problems' in N. H. Manning (ed.) *Social Problems and Welfare Ideology*, Aldershot, Hants: Gower.

Nava, M. (1988) 'Cleveland and the Press: Outrage and Anxiety in the Reporting of Child Sexual Abuse' *Feminist Review*, 28: p. 103.

Pahl, J. (1985) 'Violence against Women' in N. Manning (ed.) *Social Problems and Welfare Ideology*, Basingstoke, Hants: Gower, p. 29.

Radford, J. and Russell, D. (1992) *Femicide. The Politics of Woman Killing*, Milton Keynes, Bucks: Open University Press.

Report of the Select Committee on Violence in Marriage (1975), London: HMSO.

Russell, E. H. (1984) *Sexual Exploitation*, London: Sage.

Scott, A. (1988) 'Feminism and the Seductiveness of the "Real Event"' *Feminist Review*, 28: pp. 88–102.

Smart, C. (1989) *Feminism and the Power of Law*, London: Routledge.

—— (1992) 'The Woman of Legal Discourse' *Social and Legal Studies*, 1: p. 29.

Spector, M. and Kitsuse, J. I. (1977) *Constructing Social Problems*, New York: Aldine de Gruyter.

Spencer Brown, G. (1969) *Laws of Form*, London: Allen & Unwin.

Stets, J. E. (1988) *Domestic Violence and Control*, New York: Springer-Verlag.

Wattam, C. (1992) *Making a Case in Child Protection*, Harlow, Essex: NSPCC/Longman.

Wells, C. (1994) 'Battered Women Syndrome and Defences to Homicide: Where Now?' *Legal Studies*, 14: p. 266.

White, J. W. and Farmer, R. (1992) 'Research Methods: How They Shape Views of Sexual Violence' *Journal of Social Issues*, 48: p. 45.

Wynne, B. (1989) 'Establishing the Rules of Laws: Constructing Expert Authority' in R. Smith and B. Wynne (eds) *Expert Evidence. Interpreting Science in Law*, London and New York: Routledge, p. 23.

Wolf, N. (1993) *Fire with Fire: The New Female Power and How it Will Change the 21st Century*, London: Chatto and Windus.

CHAPTER 3 JURIDIFICATION IN THE PROTECTION OF THE SCOTTISH CHILD

Adler, R. M. (1985) *Taking Juvenile Justice Seriously*, Edinburgh: Scottish Academic Press.

Asquith, S. (1983) *Children and Justice: Decision-Making in Children's Hearings and Juvenile Courts*, Edinburgh: Edinburgh University Press.

—— (ed.) (1993) *Protecting Children. Cleveland to Orkney. More Lessons to Learn*, Edinburgh: HMSO.

Association of Directors of Social Services in Scotland (1992) *Child Protection, Policy Practice and Procedure – An Overview of Child Abuse Issues and Practice in Social Work Departments in Scotland*, Edinburgh: HMSO.

Butler-Sloss, Lord Justice (1988) *Report of the Inquiry into Child Abuse in Cleveland*, Edinburgh: HMSO.

—— (1993) 'From Cleveland to Orkney' in S. Asquith (ed.) *Protecting Children. Cleveland to Orkney. More Lessons to Learn*, Edinburgh: HMSO, pp. 53–68.

Clyde, Lord (1992) *The Report of the Inquiry into the Removal of Children from Orkney in February 1991*, Edinburgh: HMSO.

—— (1993) 'Lessons from the Orkney Inquiry' in S. Asquith (ed.) *Protecting Children. Cleveland to Orkney. More Lessons to Learn*, Edinburgh: HMSO, pp. 19–35.

Cohn, A. (1983) 'The Prevention of Child Abuse: What Do We Know About What Works?' in J. Leavitt (ed.) *Child Abuse and Neglect: Research and Innovation*, The Hague: Martinus Nijhoff.

Cooper, A. *et al.* (1995) *Positive Child Protection: A View from Abroad*, Lyme Regis, Devon: Russell House.

Dingwall, R. (1986) 'The Jasmine Beckford Affair' *Modern Law Review*, 49: pp. 488–518.

—— (1989) 'Some Problems about Predicting Child Abuse and Neglect' in O. Stevenson (ed.) *Child Abuse: Public Policy and Professional Practice*, Hemel Hempstead, Herts: Harvester-Wheatsheaf.

Duquette, D. N. (1992) 'Scottish Children's Hearings and Representation for the Child' *Justice for Children, International Conference*, Glasgow.

Fever, F. (1993) 'Long Term Abuse, Long Term Effects: a Personal Experience of Care' *Who Cares?*, reproduced in *Childright*, June, 97: p. 4.

Fletcher, G. P. (1985) 'Paradoxes in Legal Thought' *Columbia Law Review*, 25: p. 1263.

Fraser, Lord (1993) 'Legislating for Child Protection' in S. Asquith (ed.) *Protecting Children. Cleveland to Orkney. More Lessons to Learn*, Edinburgh: HMSO, pp. 37–51.

Frost, N. and Stein, M. (1989) *The Politics of Child Welfare*, Hemel Hempstead, Herts: Harvester-Wheatsheaf.

Giller, H., and Szwed, E. (1983) *Providing Civil Justice for Children*, London: Edward Arnold.

Goldstein, J., Freud, A. and Solnit, A. (1973) *Beyond the Best Interests of the Child*, New York: Free Press.

Habermas, J. (1984) *The Theory of Communicative Action, Vol. I: Reason and the Rationalization of Society*, Boston: Beacon Press.

—— (1985) 'Law as Medium and Law as Institution' in Gunther Teubner (ed.) *Dilemmas of Law in the Welfare State*, Berlin: Walter de Gruyter, pp. 203–220.

Hallett, C. (1989) 'Child Abuse Inquiries and Public Policy' in Olive Stevenson (ed.) *Child Abuse: Public Policy and Professional Practice*, Hemel Hempstead, Herts: Harvester-Wheatsheaf, pp.111–143.

Howitt, D. (1992) *Child Abuse Errors. When Good Intentions Go Wrong*, Hemel Hempstead, Herts: Harvester-Wheatsheaf.

King, M. (1991) 'Child Welfare Within Law: The Emergence of a Hybrid Discourse' *Journal of Law and Society*, 18: pp. 303–322.

—— (1993) 'The "Truth" about Autopoiesis' *Journal of Law and Society*, 20(2): pp. 1–19.

King, M. and Piper, C. (1995) *How the Law Thinks about Children*, Aldershot, Hants: Arena.

King, M. and Schütz, A. (1994) 'The Ambitious Modesty of Niklas Luhmann' *Journal of Law and Society*, 21(3): pp. 1–19.

Levy, A. and Kahan, B. (1991) *The Pindown Experience and the Protection of Children. The Report of the Staffordshire Child Care Inquiry, 1990*, Stafford: Staffordshire County Council.

Lockyer, A. (1992) 'The Scottish Children's Hearing System: Internal Developments and the UN Convention', paper given at Conference *Justice for Children*, July, Glasgow.

—— (1994) 'The Scottish Children's Hearing System: Internal Developments and the UN Convention' in S. Asquith and M. Hill (eds) *Justice for Children,* Dordrecht: Martinus Nijhoff.

Luhmann, N. (1977) 'Differentiation of Society' *Canadian Journal of Sociology*, 2(2): pp. 29–54.

—— (1985) *A Sociological Theory of Law* (2nd edn), translated by E. King and M. Albrow, London: Routledge.

—— (1988a) *The Unity of the Legal System in Autopoietic Law: A New Approach to Law and Society*, G. Teubner (ed.), Berlin and New York: Walter de Gruyter, pp.12–35.

—— (1988b) 'The Third Question: The Creative Use of Paradox in Law and Legal History' *Journal of Law and Society*, 15: pp. 153–165.

—— (1989) 'Law as a Social System' *Northwestern University Law Review*, 83: pp. 136–150.

MacIntyre, A. (1981) *After Virtue. A Study in Moral Value*, London: Duckworth.

Marshall, K. A. (1992) 'Submission to the Orkney Inquiry from the Scottish Child Law Centre', Glasgow: Scottish Child Law Centre.

Morris, A., Giller, H., Szwed, E. and Geach, H. (1980) *Justice for Children*, Basingstoke, Hants: Macmillan.

Nelken, D. (1990) 'The Truth about Law's Truth' *EUI Working Papers*, 90/1, Florence: European University Institute.

Packman, J. and Randall, J. (1989) 'Decision-making at the Gateway to Care' in O. Stevenson (ed.) *Child Abuse: Public Policy and Professional Practice*, Hemel Hempstead, Herts: Harvester-Wheatsheaf, p. 88.

Parsloe, P. (1976) 'Social Work and the Justice Model' *British Journal of Social Work*, 6: p. 72.

Parton, N. (1991) *Governing the Family. Child Care, Child Protection and the State*, Basingstoke, Hants: Macmillan.

—— (1985) *The Politics of Child Abuse*, London: Macmillan.

Preuss, U. K. (1989) 'Rational Potentials of Law: Allocative Distribution and Communicative Reality' in C. Joerges and D. Trubek (eds) *Critical Legal Thought: An Anglo-American Debate*, Baden-Baden: Nomos.

Raes, K. (1986) 'Legislation, Communication and Strategy: A Critique of Habermas' Approach to Law' *Journal of Law and Society*, 13(2): pp. 183–205.

Scottish, Child Law Centre (1993) *Response to the Social Work Services Group Consultation Paper on Emergency Protection of Children*, Glasgow: Scottish Child Law Centre.

Scottish Office Social Work Services Group (1993) *Scotland's Children:*

Proposal for Child Care Policy and Law, Scottish Office, White Paper, Cmd 2286, Edinburgh: HMSO.

Sutton, A. (1981) 'Silence in Court' in M. King (ed.) *Childhood, Welfare and Justice*, London: Batsford.

Taylor, L., Lacey, R. and Bracken, D. (1979) *In Whose Best Interests?*, London: Cobden Trust/Mind.

Teubner, G. (1989) 'How the Law Thinks: Toward a Constructivist Epistomology of Law' *Law and Society Review*, 23: pp. 727–757.

—— (1992) *Law as an Autopoietic System*, Oxford: Blackwell.

Thane, P. (1981) 'Childhood in History.' in M. King (ed.) *Childhood, Welfare and Justice*, London: Batsford, pp. 6–25.

Wallerstein, J. and Kelly, J. (1981) *Surviving the Break-up*, New York: Grant McIntyre.

Wroe, A. (1988) *Social Work, Child Abuse and the Press*, Norwich: University of East Anglia.

CHAPTER 4 DOING GOOD FOR CHILDREN – MISSION IMPOSSIBLE?

The Audit Commission (1986) *Performance Review in Local Government. A Handbook for Auditors and Local Authorities*, London: HMSO.

—— (1994) *Seen But Not Heard*, London: HMSO.

Baecker, D. (1994) 'Sociale Hilfe als Funktionssystem der Gesellshaft' *Zeitshrift für Soziologie*, 23: p. 93.

Brown, P. (1993) *The Captured World*, Hemel Hempstead, Herts: Harvester-Wheatsheaf.

Clarke, J., Cochrane, A. and McLaughlin, E. (eds) (1994) *Managing Social Policy*, London: Sage.

Cooper, A. et al. (1995) *Positive Child Protection: A View from Abroad*, Lyme Regis, Devon: Russell House.

DHSS (1982) *Child Abuse: A Study of Inquiry Reports 1973–1981*, London: HMSO.

DHSS Inspectorate (1993) *Inspecting for Quality. Evaluating Performance in Child Protection. A Framework for the Inspection of Local Authority Social Services Practice and Systems*, London: HMSO.

—— (1995) *The Challenge of Partnership in Child Protection: Practice Guide*, London: HMSO.

Foucault, M. (1977) *Discipline and Punish*, London: Allen Lane.

—— (1978) 'About the Concept of the "Dangerous Individual" in 19th-Century Legal Psychiatry' *International Journal of Law and Psychiatry*, 1–18.

—— (1979) *The History of Sexuality, Vol I: An Introduction*, London: Allen Lane.

Garland, D. (1985) *Punishment and Welfare. A History of Penal Strategies*, Aldershot, Hants: Gower.

Halmos, P. (1965) *The Faith of the Counsellors*, London: Constable.

—— (1966) 'The Personal Service Society', Inaugural Lecture, University College Cardiff.

Hodges, J. and Hussein, A. (1979) 'Review of Donzelot' *Ideology and Consciousness*, 5.

Home Office, Department of Health, Department of Education and Science (1991) *Working Together under the Children Act 1989*, London: HMSO.

Howe, D. (1992) 'Child Abuse and the Bureaucratisation of Social Work' *The Sociological Review*, 40: pp. 491–508.

Howitt, D. (1992) *Child Abuse Errors. When Good Intentions go Wrong*, Hemel Hempstead, Herts: Harvester-Wheatsheaf.

Johnson, T. J. (1972) *Professions and Power*, London: Macmillan.

King, M. (1995) 'Law's Healing of Children's Hearings. The Paradox Moves North' *Journal of Social Policy*, 24: pp. 1–26.

King, M. and Piper, C. (1995) *How the Law Thinks about Children* (2nd edn), Aldershot, Hants: Arena.

Kroll, B. (1995) 'Working in Partnership with Children' in F. Kaganas, M. King and C. Piper (eds) *Legislating for Harmony. Partnership under the Children Act*, London: Jessica Kingsley.

Langan, M. and Clarke, J. C. (1994) 'Managing in the Mixed Economy of Care' in J. Clarke, A. Cochrane and E. McLaughlin (eds) *Managing Social Policy*, London: Sage.

Luhmann, N. (1977) 'Differentiation of Society' *Canadian Journal of Sociology*, 2(2): pp. 29–54.

—— (1982) 'The World Society as a Social System' *International Journal of General Systems*, 8: pp. 131–138.

—— (1986a) 'The Autopoiesis of Social Systems' in F. Geyer and J. van der Zouwen (eds) *Sociocybernetic Paradoxes: Observation, Control and Evolution of Self-Steering Systems*, pp. 171–192.

—— (1986b) 'The Theory of Social Systems and its Epistemology: Reply to Danilo Zolo's Critical Comments' *Philosophy of the Social Sciences*, 16: pp. 112–131

—— (1987) 'The Representation of Society within Society' *Current Sociology*, 35: pp. 101–108.

—— (1989) *Ecological Communications*, Chicago: University of Chicago Press.

—— (1990) *Essays on Self Reference*, New York: Columbia University Press.

—— (1993) *Risk: A Sociological Theory*, New York: Aldine de Gruyter.

Pahl, J. (1994) '"Like the Job, but Hate the Organisation". Social Workers and Managers in Social Services' *Social Policy Review*, 6: p. 190.

Parton, N. (1991) *Governing the Family. Child Care, Child Protection and the State*, Basingstoke, Hants: Macmillan.

Philp, M. (1979) 'Notes on the Form of Knowledge in Social Work' *Sociological Review*, 27: pp. 83–111.

Platt, A. M. (1969) *The Child Savers: The Invention of Delinquency*, Chicago: Chicago University Press.

Pollitt, C. (1990) *Managerialism and the Public Services. The Anglo-American Experience*, Oxford: Blackwell.

Pollitt, C. and Harrison, S. (eds) (1992) *Handbook of Public Service Management*, Oxford: Blackwell.

Poynter, J. R. (1969) *Society and Pauperism. English Ideas on Poor Relief 1795–1834'*, London: Routledge and Kegan Paul.

Valentine, M. (1994) 'The Social Worker as Bad Object' *British Journal of Social Work*, 24: p. 749.

Wynne, B. (1989) 'Establishing the Rules of Laws: Constructing Expert Authority' in R. Smith and B. Wynne (eds) *Expert Evidence. Interpreting Science in Law*, London and New York: Routledge, pp. 23–55.

CHAPTER 5 THE JAMES BULGER TRIAL: GOOD OR BAD FOR GUILTY OR INNOCENT CHILDREN?

Asquith, S. (1996) 'When Children Kill Children. The Search for Justice' *The Childhood Journal*, 3(1).

Cohen, S. (1980) *Folk Devils and Moral Panic*, London: MacGibbon and Kee.

Garland, D. (1988) *Punishment and Welfare. A History of Penal Strategies* Aldershot, Hants: Gower.

Geertz, C. (1983) *Local Knowledge. Further Essays in Interpretive Anthropology*, New York: Basic Books.

Hall, S. E. A. (1978) *Policing the Crisis: Mugging, the State and Law-and-Order*, London: Macmillan.

Hay, C. (1995) 'Mobilization through Interpellation' *Social and Legal Studies*, 4: p. 197.

King, M. and Piper, C. (1995) *How the Law Thinks about Children* (2nd edn), Aldershot, Hants: Arena.

King, M. and Schütz, A. (1994) 'The Ambitious Modesty of Niklas Luhmann' *Journal of Law and Society*, 21(3): p. 261.

Luhmann, N. (1989) *Ecological Communications*, Chicago: University of Chicago Press

—— (1992) 'Operational Closure and Structural Coupling: The Differentiation of the Legal System' *Cardozo Law Review*, 13: pp. 1419–1441.

—— (1993) *Risk: A Sociological Theory* (translated by R. Barrett), Berlin and New York: Walter de Gruyter.

Sereny G. (1994) 'Re-examining the Evidence' *Independent Magazine*, 8 February: pp. 4–10; and 'Establishing the Truth' 13 February: pp. 5–9.

Smith, D. J. (1994) *The Sleep of Reason. The James Bulger Case*, London: Century.

Smith, K. J. M. (1988) *James Fitzjames Stephen. Portrait of a Victorian Rationalist*, Oxford: Oxford University Press.

Stephen, J. F. (1883) *History of the Criminal Law of England*, Vol. II, London: Macmillan.

CHAPTER 6   REAL AND IMAGINED COMMUNITIES AND FAMILIES

Adler, C. and Wundersitz, J. (1994) *Family Conferencing and Juvenile Justice*, Canberra, Australia: Australian Institute of Criminology.

Anderson, B. (1991) *Imagined Communities. Reflections on the Origin and Spread of Nationalism* (2nd edn), London: Verso.

Ashenden, S. (1995) 'Political Rationality and Child Sexuality' in   A. Barry, N. Rose and V. Bell (eds) *Liberalism, Neo-Liberalism and the Rationality of Government*, London: UCL Press.

Atkin, W. R. (1988–1989) 'New Zealand: Children Versus Families – Is there a Conflict?.' *Journal of Family Law*, p. 231.

Beck, U. (1992) *Risk Society*, London: Sage.

Braithwaite, J. (1992) 'Juvenile Offending: Theory and Practice' in L. Atkinson and S.-A. Gerull (eds) *National Conference on Juvenile Justice: 22–24 September 1992*, Canberra: Australian Institute of Criminology.

—— (1993) 'Inequality and Republican Criminology' in J. Hagan and R. D. Peterson (eds) *Crime and Inequality*, Palo Alto, Cal.: Stanford University Press.

—— (1994) 'Thinking Harder about Democratising Social Control' in C. Adler and J. Wundersitz (eds) Family Conferencing and Juvenile Justice, Canberra, Australia: Australian Institute of Criminology.

Braithwaite, J. and Mugford, S. (1994) 'Conditions of Successful Reintegration Ceremonies' *British Journal of Criminology*, 34: pp.139–170.

Braithwaite, J. and Petit, P. (1990) *Not Just Deserts: A Republican Theory of Criminal Justice*, Oxford: Oxford University Press.

Calhoun, C. (1994) 'Social Theory and the Politics of Identity' in C. Calhoun (ed.) *Social Theory and the Politics of Identity*, Oxford: Blackwell.

Department of Social Welfare (1987) *Report of the Working Party on the Children and Young Persons Bill*, Wellington, New Zealand: Department of Social Welfare.

Freeman, M. (1994) 'Protecting Children on Both sides of the Globe' *Adelaide Law Review*, 16: p. 79.

King, M. and Trowell, J. (1992) *Children's Welfare and the Law. The Limits of Legal Intervention*, London: Sage.

Luhmann, N. (1993) *Risk: A Sociological Theory*, New York: Aldine de Gruyter.

Lupton, C., Barnard, S. and Swall-Yarrington, M. (1995) *Family Planning?: An Evaluation of the Family Group Conference Model*, Portsmouth: Social Service Research and Information Unit, University of Portsmouth.

Manning, N. (1985) 'Constructing Social Problems' in N. H. Manning (ed.) *Social Problems and Welfare Ideology*, Aldershot, Hants: Gower.

Moore, D. (1992) 'Facing the Consequences' in L. Atkinson and S.-A. Gerull (eds) *National Conference on Juvenile Justice*, Canberra: Australian Institute of Criminology.

Polk, K. (1994) 'Family Conferencing, Theoretical and Evaluative

Concerns' in C. Adler and J. Wundersitz (eds) *Family Conferencing and Juvenile Justice*, Canberra, Australia: Australian Institute of Criminology.

Piper, C. (1993) *The Responsible Parent. A Study in Divorce Mediation*, Hemel Hempstead, Herts: Harvester-Wheatsheaf.

Sandor, D. (1994) 'The Thickening Blue Wedge' in C. Adler and J. Wundersitz (eds) *Family Conferencing and Juvenile Justice*, Canberra, Australia: Australian Institute of Criminology.

Spector, M. and Kitsuse, J. I. (1977) *Constructing Social Problems*, New York: Aldine de Gruyter.

Stainton Rogers, R. and W. (1992) *Stories of Childhood. Shifting Agendas of Child Concern*, Hemel Hempstead, Herts: Harvester-Wheatsheaf.

Swain, D. (1995) 'Family Group Conferences in Child Care and Protection and in Youth Justice in Aotearoa/New Zealand' *International Journal of Law and the Family*, 9: p. 155.

Webb, P. R. (1992) *Family Law in New Zealand* (5th edn), Wellington, New Zealand: Butterworths.

White, R. (1994) 'Shame and Integration Strategies: Individuals, State Power and Social Interests' in C. Adler and J. Wundersitz (eds) *Family Conferencing and Juvenile Justice*, Canberra, Australia: Australian Institute of Criminology

CHAPTER 7 OBSERVING CHILDREN'S RIGHTS

Alston, P. (1994) 'The Best Interests Principle: Towards a Reconciliation of Culture and Human Rights' *International Journal of Law and the Family*, 8: p. 1.

Alston, P., Parker, S. and Seymour, J. (1992) *Children, Rights and the Law*, Oxford: Clarendon.

Beck, U. (1992) *Risk Society*, London: Sage.

Berger, P. and Luckmann, T. (1966) *The Social Construction of Reality: A Treatise in the Sociology of Knowledge*, New York: Doubleday.

Boydon, J. (1990) 'Childhood and the Policy Makers: A Comparative Study on the Globalization of Childhood' in A. James and A. Prout (eds) *Reconstructing Childhood: Contemporary Issues in the Sociological Study of Childhood*, London: Farmer, p. 184.

Catterall, C. D. (1980) 'The Declaration of the Psychological Rights of the Child' *Association of Educational Psychologists Journal*, p. 34.

Cohen, C. P. (1990) 'The Role of Nongovernmental Organizations in the Drafting of the Convention on the Rights of the Child' *Human Rights Quarterly*, 12: pp. 137–147.

Crowe, R. (1995) 'Trolley full of Empties' *The Guardian*, 8 August.

Fairchild, H. N. (1928) *The Noble Savage*, New York: Columbia University Press.

Freeman, M. (1995) 'The Morality of Cultural Pluralism' *The International Journal of Children's Rights*, 3: p. 1.

Jenks, C. (1996) *Childhood*, London: Routledge

King, M. (1982) 'Children's Rights in Education: More than a Slogan?' *Educational Studies*, 8: pp. 227–238.

—— (1993) 'The "Truth" about Autopoiesis' *Journal of Law and Society*, 20(2): pp. 1–19.

—— (1994) 'Children's Rights as Communication' *Modern Law Review*, 57(3): pp. 385–401.

—— (1995a) *God's Law versus State Law: The Construction of an Islamic Identity in Western Europe*, London: Grey Seal.

—— (1995b) 'Religion into Law, Law into Religion: the Construction of a Secular Identity for Islam' in P. Fitzpatrick (ed.) *Nationalism, Racism and the Rule of Law*, Aldershot, Hants: Dartmouth, p. 167

King, M. and Schütz, A. (1994) 'The Ambitious Modesty of Niklas Luhmann' *Journal of Law and Society*, 21(3): pp. 261–287.

Kroll, B. (1994) *Chasing Rainbows: Children, Divorce and Loss*, Lyme Regis, Devon: Russell House.

—— (1995) 'Working with Children' in F. Kaganas, M. King and C. Piper (eds) *Legislating for Harmony. Partnership under the Children Act, 1995*, London: Jessica Kingsley.

Luhmann, N. (1977) 'Differentiation of Society' *Canadian Journal of Sociology*, 2(2): pp. 29–54.

—— (1982) 'The World Society as a Social System' *International Journal of General Systems*, 8(8): pp. 131–138.

—— (1985) *A Sociological Theory of Law* (2nd edn), London: Routledge.

—— (1986) 'The Individuality of the Individual: Historical Meanings and Contemporary Problems' in T. Heller, M. Sosna and D. E. Wellbery (eds) *Restructuring Individualism: Autonomy, Individuality and the Self in Western Thought*, Palo Alto, Cal.: Stanford University Press, p. 313.

—— (1988) 'The Unity of the Legal System' in G. Teubner (ed.) *Autopoietic Law: A New Approach to Law and Society Berlin*, New York: Walter de Gruyter.

—— (1989a) 'Law as a Social System' *Northwestern University Law Review*, 83(1 & 2): pp. 136–150.

—— (1989b) *Wirtschaft und Recht: Probleme strucktureller Kopplung*, Bielefeld: Manuskript.

—— (1990) *Political Theory in the Welfare State*, Berlin and New York: Walter de Gruyter.

—— (1992) 'Operational Closure and Structural Coupling: The Differentiation of the Legal System' *Cardozo Law Review*, 13: pp. 1419–1441.

—— (1993) 'The Code of the Moral' *Cardozo Law Review*, 14: pp. 995–1009.

Mead, G. H. (1934) *Mind, Self and Society: From the Standpoint of a Social Behaviourist*, Chicago: University of Chicago Press.

Teubner, G. (1992) 'Social Order from Legislative Noise? Autopoietic Closure as a Problem for Legal Regulation' in G. Teubner and A. Febbrajo (eds) *European Yearbook of the Sociology of Law*, Milan: Giuffrè.

—— (1993) Law as an Autopoietic System, Oxford: Blackwell.

CHAPTER 8 A DIFFERENT WORLD FOR CHILDREN

Archard, D. (1993) *Children, Rights and Childhood*, London: Routledge.
Ariès, P. (1962) *Centuries of Childhood*, London: Jonathan Cape.
Beck, U. (1992) *Risk Society*, London: Sage.
Boydon, J. (1990) 'Childhood and the Policy Makers: A Comparative Study on the Globalization of Childhood' in A. James and A. Prout (eds) *Reconstructing Childhood: Contemporary Issues in the Sociological Study of Childhood*, London: Farmer, p. 184.
Hegel, G. W. F. (1977) *The Phenomenology of Spirit*, Oxford: Oxford University Press.
Hobson, D. (1995) 'State of the Argument' *Prospect*, 1: p. 8.
King, M. and Piper, C. (1995) *How the Law Thinks about Children* (2nd edn), Aldershot, Hants: Arena.
King, M. and Trowell, J. (1992) *Children's Welfare and the Law: The Limits of Legal Intervention*, London: Sage.
Teubner, G. (in press) 'Altera pars audiatur. Law in the Collision of Discourses' in R. Rawlings (ed.) *Law, Society and Economy*, Oxford: Oxford University Press.
Wynne, B. (1989) 'Establishing the Rules of Laws: Constructing Expert Authority' in Roger Smith and Brian Wynne (eds) *Expert Evidence. Interpreting Science in Law*, pp. 23–55.

Name index

Subject index

abuse *see* child abuse
adult/child distinction 3–4, 169–70, 171, 185, 193, 195–7
anti-child abuse campaigns; and economics 52–4; feminist inspired 36–40; and law 44–8; as perturbations for social systems 42–54; and politics 48–52; and science 43–4; *see also* child abuse
Australia, family group conference project in 147–52, 159
authority 30; fragmentation of 15–19, 20, 35; and regulation 11–15, 17
autopoietic systems 92, 152, 173–7, 180, 183–4, 199–200; and authority discourses 27; as closed 173–7; communications with 26–8; complexity 28, 57; contingency 28; people and society as 26; *see also* autopoietic theory; social systems, closed systems
autopoietic theory 26–9, 42, 102, 122, 147, 153–4, 177, 179, 180, 189; *see also* autopoietic systems; social systems

behaviour 142; explanations of 63;

interpretation of 43–4; legal view of 175
benefits *see* harms and benefits
Bulger, James, murder 109–29; and search for causes 121–2, 128

caring professions, emergence of 88–91
chance, and foreseeability 22–4
child abuse 1–2, 5, 22, 29, 92, 143–4, 147, 194; and certainty of uncertainty 54–5; and child removal from the home 62–3; clear evidence for 74–5; identification/prediction of 64–5; interpretation of 64; and male power 32, 37–9; monistic explanations of 100; remedies for 40–2; survivors of 185; *see also* anti-child abuse campaigns
Child Advocate 79, 85
child labour 176, 180–2
child protection agencies 60
child welfare 2, 51, 67–8, 69, 75, 77, 98–9, 127, 153–4, 197; paradox of 61–7; *see also* welfare
childhood 63, 67, 116, 127–8, 164, 168, 172, 192, 197
children, devaluing of 117; future